AF413075

Clinical Management of Soft Tissue Sarcomas

Cancer Treatment and Research

WILLIAM L MCGUIRE, *series editor*

Livingston RB (ed): Lung Cancer 1. 1981. ISBN 90-247-2394-9.
Bennett Humphrey G, Dehner LP, Grindey GB, Acton RT (eds): Pediatric Oncology 1. 1981. ISBN 90-247-2408-2.
DeCosse JJ, Sherlock P (eds): Gastrointestinal Cancer 1. 1981. ISBN 90-247-2461-9.
Bennett JM (ed): Lymphomas 1, including Hodgkin's Disease. 1981. ISBN 90-247-2479-1.
Bloomfield CD (ed): Adult Leukemias 1. 1982. ISBN 90-247-2478-3.
Paulson DF (ed): Genitourinary Cancer 1. 1982. ISBN 90-247-2480-5.
Muggia FM (ed): Cancer Chemotherapy 1. ISBN 90-247-2713-8.
Bennett Humphrey G, Grindey GB (eds): Pancreatic Tumors in Children. 1982. ISBN 90-247-2702-2.
Costanzi JJ (ed): Malignant Melanoma 1. 1983. ISBN 90-247-2706-5.
Griffiths CT, Fuller AF (eds): Gynecologic Oncology. 1983. ISBN 0-89838-555-5.
Greco AF (ed): Biology and Management of Lung Cancer. 1983. ISBN 0-89838-554-7.
Walker MD (ed): Oncology of the Nervous System. 1983. ISBN 0-89838-567-9.
Higby DJ (ed): Supportive Care in Cancer Therapy. 1983. ISBN 0-89838-569-5.
Herberman RB (ed): Basic and Clinical Tumor Immunology. 1983. ISBN 0-89838-579-2.
Baker LH (ed): Soft Tissue Sarcomas. 1983. ISBN 0-89838-584-9.
Bennett JM (ed): Controversies in the Management of Lymphomas. 1983. ISBN 0-89838-586-5.
Bennett Humphrey G, Grindey GB (eds): Adrenal and Endocrine Tumors in Children. 1983. ISBN 0-89838-590-3.
DeCosse JJ, Sherlock P (eds): Clinical Management of Gastrointestinal Cancer. 1984. ISBN 0-89838-601-2.
Catalona WJ, Ratliff TL (eds): Urologic Oncology. 1984. ISBN 0-89838-628-4.
Santen RJ, Manni A (eds): Diagnosis and Management of Endocrine-related Tumors. 1984. ISBN 0-89838-636-5.
Costanzi JJ (ed): Clinical Management of Malignant Melanoma. 1984. ISBN 0-89838-656-X.
Wolf GT (ed): Head and Neck Oncology. 1984. ISBN 0-89838-657-8.
Alberts DS, Surwit EA (eds): Ovarian Cancer. 1985. ISBN 0-89838-676-4.
Muggia FM (ed): Experimental and Clinical Progress in Cancer Chemotherapy. 1985. ISBN 0-89838-679-9.
Higby DJ (ed): The Cancer Patient and Supportive Care. 1985. ISBN 0-89838-690-X.
Bloomfield CD (ed): Chronic and Acute Leukemias in Adults. 1985. ISBN 0-89838-702-7.
Herberman RB (ed): Cancer Immunology: Innovative Approaches to Therapy. 1986. ISBN 0-89838-757-4.
Hansen HH (ed): Lung Cancer: Basic and Clinical Aspects. 1986. ISBN 0-89838-763-9.
Pinedo HM, Verweij J (eds): Clinical Management of Soft Tissue Sarcomas. 1986. ISBN 0-89838-808-2.
Higby DJ (ed): Issues in Supportive Care of Cancer Patients. 1986. ISBN 0-89838-816-3.

Clinical Management of Soft Tissue Sarcomas

edited by

H.M. PINEDO
Department of Oncology
Free University Hospital
De Boelelaan 1117
1081 HV Amsterdam, The Netherlands

and

J. VERWEIJ
Department of Oncology
The Dr. Daniel den Hoed Cancer Center
Groene Hilledijk 301
3075 EA Rotterdam, The Netherlands

1986 **MARTINUS NIJHOFF PUBLISHERS** 
a member of the KLUWER ACADEMIC PUBLISHERS GROUP
BOSTON / DORDRECHT / LANCASTER

Distributors

for the United States and Canada: Kluwer Academic Publishers, 101 Philip Drive, Assinippi Park, Norwell, MA 02061, USA
for the UK and Ireland: Kluwer Academic Publishers, MTP Press Limited, Falcon House, Queen Square, Lancaster LA1 1RN, UK
for all other countries: Kluwer Academic Publishers Group, Distribution Center, P.O. Box 322, 3300 AH Dordrecht, The Netherlands

Library of Congress Cataloging in Publication Data

```
Clinical management of soft tissue sarcomas.

  (Cancer treatment and research ; CTAR 29)
  Includes bibliographies and index.
  1. Sarcoma.  I Pinedo, H. M.  II. Verweij, J. (Jaap)
III. Series.  [DNLM: 1. Sarcoma--diagnosis.  2. Sarcoma
--therapy.  W1 CA693 v.29 / QZ 345 C641]
RC262.C534  1986      616.99'4          86-8339
ISBN 0-89838-808-2
```

ISBN 0-89838-808-2 (this volume)
ISBN 90-247-2426-0 (series)

Copyright

Table of Contents

Cancer Treatment and Research

Foreword

Where do you begin to look for a recent, authoritative article on the diagnosis or management of a particular malignancy? The few general oncology textbooks are generally out of date. Single papers in specialized journals are informative but seldom comprehensive; these are more often preliminary reports on a very limited number of patients. Certain general journals frequently publish good indepth reviews of cancer topics, and published symposium lectures are often the best overviews available. Unfortunately, these reviews and supplements appear sporadically, and the reader can never be sure when a topic of special interest will be covered.

Cancer Treatment and Research is a series of authoritative volumes which aim to meet this need. It is an attempt to establish a critical mass of oncology literature covering virtually all oncology topics, revised frequently to keep the coverage up to date, easily available on a single library shelf or by a single personal subscription.

We have approached the problem in the following fashion. First, by dividing the oncology literature into specific subdivisions such as lung cancer, genitourinary cancer, pediatric oncology, etc. Second, by asking eminent authorities in each of these areas to edit a volume on the specific topic on an annual or biannual basis. Each topic and tumor type is covered in a volume appearing frequently and predictably, discussing current diagnosis, staging, markers, all forms of treatment modalities, basic biology, and more.

In Cancer Treatment and Research, we have an outstanding group of editors, each having made a major commitment to bring to this new series the very best literature in his or her field. Martinus Nijhoff Publishers has made an equally major commitment to the rapid publication of high quality books, and world-wide distribution.

Where can you go to find quickly a recent authoritative article on any major oncology problem? We hope that Cancer Treatment and Research provides an answer.

WILLIAM L. MCGUIRE
Series Editor

Preface

Although soft tissue sarcomas are rare tumors, representing only ±1% of all malignant tumors in adults, they remain a challenge to all disciplines in medical treatment and research. Apart from research in all fields of treatment, soft tissue sarcomas are also encountered in several forms of combined modality treatment.

Since the appearance of the first volume on soft tissue sarcomas in this series (*Soft Tissue Sarcomas*, Laurence H. Baker, ed., Martinus Nijhoff Publishers, 1983), a large amount of data has emerged from preclinical as well as clinical investigations. The present volume provides an up-to-date review of the state of the art without duplicating the contents of the earlier volume.

In the chapter on pathology it is again indicated that malignant fibrocytic hystiocytoma is at present the most frequently diagnosed type of soft tissue sarcoma. Nevertheless, sub-typing is less important for the prognosis than grade. Recently, grading has been defined better, permitting a more common use of this prognostic factor. However, the experience of the pathologist is most important for adequate grading. The pathologist will need an adequate biopsy to perform his investigations. Cytology is not sufficient for diagnosis. However, for confirmation of metastatic lesions, cytology may provide enough information. Some new tools have been added to the equipment of the pathologist.

Electronmicroscopy appears to be a useful technique in classifying previously so-called undifferentiated sarcomas. Special histochemical markers such as cytokeratins, vimentin, desmin, neurofilament protein and glial fibrillary acidic protein are also useful in the typing of soft tissue sarcomas. Once a diagnosis has been made, further staging will be important in order to assure adequate treatment. Soft tissue sarcomas frequently metastasize to the lungs. Tomography or CT-scanning of the lungs will reveal an important number of lung metastasis in patients previously considered as having local disease. For further evaluation of the local tumor mass CT-scan may provide reliable information on the transverse extent of the tumor. The role of nuclear magnetic resonance has yet to be defined. Bone scanning play a dual role in the diagnostics of soft tissue sarcomas.

With the information obtained by diagnostic techniques, we may adequately stage the patient with a soft tissue sarcoma. Because of the excellent correlations with survival, the staging system of the American Joint Committee is preferred. It is based on the TMM-classification, but also includes grade. Other staging systems will not be as reliable concerning prognosis.

Surgery is still the only chance for cure in soft tissue sarcomas. It is of utmost importance to direct the incision so that the biopsy site, as well as those underlying structures that have to be removed, are included. Furthermore, the incision should be directed along the pathway for metastases. Truncal lesions require wide resection with adequate marging of surrounding normal tissue, sometimes necessitating resection of parts of the chest- or abdominal wall, in which case a marlex mesh may increase stability. For extremity lesions the results of limb saving procedures are equal to those of amputation, as far as recurrence and survival are concerned. Therefore, amputation should be avoided if possible. Wide resection with muscle group dissection, followed by local radiotherapy, results in an adequate function of the extremity without decreasing survival.

The value of radiotherapy in limb saving procedures is well recognized, but besides there appears to be a considerable change in the role of radiotherapy in the treatment of soft tissue sarcomas. Radiotherapy as part of combined modalities enjoys a revived interest as indicated by studies on preoperative radiotherapy, interstitial radiotherapy, intraoperative radiotherapy for retroperitoneal sarcomas, and in combination with radiosensitizers. Radiotherapy alone may achieve a 30% local control in inoperable tumors.

Concerning chemotherapy some important conclusions have been drawn in the past few years. For the treatment of disseminated disease, combination chemotherapy appears to result in higher response rates than single agent treatment. The combination of cyclophosphamide, vincristine, doxorubicin and dacarbazine (CYVADIC) results in both the highest total response rate as well as the highest complete response rate. Although this regimen has not been compared to the second best regimen, doxorubicin plus dacarbazine (ADIC), the higher complete response rate of CYVADIC is still a good reason to select this regimen as standard therapy for patients in a good condition.

After a period of silence, a new active drug in the treatment of soft tissue sarcomas has been discovered in the recent years. This drug is ifosfamide, which in several trials appears to be much more active than Cyclophosphamide, and achieves a response rate of approximately 20%, which approaches that of doxorubicin. The combination of doxorubicin and ifosfamide is attractive for further studies. Preliminary data show a response rate of 35–40%. The usefulness of adjuvant chemotherapy has been questioned more and more. Most of the trials concerning this type of treatment have been non-randomized and suggest a benefit for the patient. More recently several randomized trials with a control group have been initiated. At present, with one exception, they do not show any benefit of adjuvant chemotherapy. All are subject to criticism concerning incompleteness. This also holds for the preliminary results of the largest randomized trial, conducted by the EORTC. For this reason adjuvant chemotherapy should not be considered standard treatment for soft tissue sarcomas at this time. In case of locally advanced but non-metastatic disease, especially when the tumor is located in the extremities, intraarterial infusion or perfusion may lead to interesting results.

Intraarterial chemotherapy may achieve tumor reduction permitting less extensive surgery and also gives an indication of tumor responsiveness to the chemotherapy given, which may be important for studies on adjuvant chemotherapy. However, the results available for the moment do not indicate any survival improvement of the patients treated. An important fact appears to be the absence of major complications of catheterisations when performed by experienced physicians. This is an improvement, compared to previous studies using this type of treatment. Another important fact is that the absence of measurable tumor shrinkage does not predict for histological response; even in the absence of tumor reduction microscopic investigations may indicate major tumor necroses. The use of hyperthermic antiblastic perfusion in locally advanced disease is a new exciting development. However, it should still be considered investigational and the results are too preliminary to draw definite conclusions.

This volume extensively discusses all of these topics. For all chapters, authoritive authors from all over the world have contributed, and we would like to thank them for their kind cooperation.

May this book ultimately be of benefit for the patient.

H. M. Pinedo, J. Verweij,
editors

List of contributors

SALVATORE ANDREOLA M.D., Dept. of Pathology, Instituto Nazionale per lo Studio e la Cura dei Tumori, Via Venezian 1, 20133 Milan, Italy.

MYRON ARLEN M.D., Dept. of Surgery, North Shore University Hospital, 300 Community Drive, Manhasset, New York 11030, United States of America.

ALBERTO AZZARELLI M.D., Dept. of Surgical Oncology, Instituto Nazionale per lo Studio e la Cura dei tumori, Via Venezian 1, 20133 Milan, Italy.

VIVIAN H. D. BRAMWELL M.B., B.S., M.R.C.P., Dept. of Medical Oncology, London Regional Cancer Center, 391 South Street, London, Ontario N6A 4G5, Canada.

LEONARDO GENNARI M.D., Dept. of Surgical Oncology, Instituto Nazionale per lo Studio e la Cura dei Tumori, Via Venezian 1, 20133 Milan, Italy.

ELI J. GLATSTEIN M.D., Radiation Oncology Branch, Division of Cancer Treatment NCI, Bethesda MD 20205, United States of America.

JANE GRAYSON M.D., Radiation Oncology Branch, Division of Cancer Treatment NCI, Bethesda MD 20205, United States of America.

RALPH C. MARCOVE M.D., Dept. of Surgery, Memorial Sloan Kettering Cancer Center, 1275 York Avenue, New York, NY 10021, United States of America.

DAVID E. MARKHAM F.R.C.S., Dept. of Surgery, Manchester Royal Infirmary, Oxford Road, Manchester M13 9WL, United Kingdom.

ALLN T. VAN OOSTEROM M.D., Dept. of Medical Oncology, State University Hospital, Rijnsburgerweg 233, 2333 AA Leiden, The Netherlands.

HERBERT M. PINEDO M.D., Dept. of Medical Oncology, Free University Hospital, De Boelelaan 1117, 1081 HV Amsterdam, The Netherlands.

MARIO SANTINAMI M.D., Dept. of Surgical Oncology, Instituto Nazionale per lo Studio e la Cura dei Tumori, Via Venezian 1, 20133 Milan, Italy.

GEORGE A. TRIVETTE M.D., Radiation Oncology Branch, Division of Cancer Treatment NCI, Bethesda MD 20205, United States of America.

AD J. M. VAN UNNIK M.D., Dept. of Pathology, Grootziekengasthuis, Nieuwstraat 34, 5211 NL Den Bosch, The Netherlands.

JAN A. M. VAN UNNIK M.D., Dept. of Pathology, State University Hospital,

Catharijnesingel 101, 3583 CP Utrecht, The Netherlands.
MAURIZO VAGLINI M.D., Dept. of Surgical Oncology, Instituto Nazionale per lo Studio e la Cura dei Tumori, Via Venezian 1, 20133 Milan, Italy.
JAAP VERWEIJ, M.D., Dept. of Medical Oncology, Dr. Daniel den Hoed Cancer Center, Groene Hilledijk 301, 3075 EA Rotterdam, The Netherlands.

List of abbreviatons

AMPB	=	Amphotericin B
CDDP	=	Cisplatin
CLB	=	Chloorambucil
CTX	=	Cyclophosphamide
DACT	=	Actinomycin D
DTIC	=	Dimethyl Trianzino Immidazole Carboxamide
DX	=	Doxorubicine
IFX	=	Ifosfamide
Me-CCNU	=	Methyl-CCNU
MTX	=	Methotrexate
VCR	=	Vincristine
VDS	=	Vindesine

1. Pathology of soft tissue sarcomas

J. A. M. van Unnik and A. J. M. van Unnik

Introduction

The increase in therapeutic modalities for soft tissue sarcomas requires an optimal histopathological categorization of these malignancies. Only in this way the clinician is provided with a reliable prediction of the behaviour of a particular lesion. Moreover a strict definition of these entities and a high degree of reproducibility is a prerequisite for a comparison of therapeutic results which forms a basis for further progress in this field. Only a better understanding of the histogenesis of these malignancies provides a starting point for the delineation of the different categories. In the past decades additional techniques such as electron microscopy and the use of immunohistochemical markers have extended our diagnostic tools, but at the same time they have questioned time-honoured conceptions.

The histopathologic typing of malignancies in general and soft tissue sarcomas in particular has to be supplemented by a grading system to obtain more information from the histopathological examination. Soft tissue sarcomas in contrast to organ specific tumors may originate in widely different locations. It has become apparent that these differences in location may influence, sometimes to a high degree, the prognosis of these lesions. For the planning of a surgical resection one needs some knowledge about the mode of infiltration. Some soft tissue sarcomas are notorious in this respect e.g. myxoid liposarcomas which may have imperceptible extensions and malignant schwannomas which may spread along peripheral nerves. The aforementioned prognostic indicators are completed by the staging of the disease [1], in which the pathologist may contribute by giving the exact size of the tumor and the histopathological diagnosis of lesions suspect for secondaries.

The term soft tissue tumor is rather vague. In no other field of oncology is the consistency of the tissue of origin the only quality used to designate a group of malignancies. Hence it is appropriate to present a brief definition of these tumors as originally outlined in the soft tissue classification of the World Health Organization [2]. 'Soft tissue sarcomas are comprised of all malignant tumors of non-

Pinedo, H. M., Verweij, J (eds) Clinical Management of Soft Tissue Sarcomas
© *1986 Martinus Nijhoff Publishers, Boston. ISBN 0-89838-808-2. Printed in The Netherlands.*

2

epithelial, extraskeletal tissues with the exception of the hematopoietic system, glia and supporting tissues of specific organs and viscera. Malignant tumors of the peripheral and autonomic nervous system are included among the soft tissue sarcomas because they pose similar problems in diagnosis and therapy.'

Aetiology

In contrast to epithelial malignancies no obvious causative agents are known in the majority of soft tissue sarcomas. Congenital-familial factors can be assigned in some types of sarcomas. Recklinghausen's disease means a notorious predisposition for the occurrence of soft tissue sarcomas especially neurogenic sarcomas [3]. The cancer family syndrome involves soft tissue sarcomas in children and early onset cancers in close relatives especially breast cancer in the mother [4, 5] also rhabdomyosarcomas may be associated with neurofibromatosis [6] and the basal cell nevus syndrome [7].

A viral origin for human sarcomas is still a matter of dispute. The occurrence of Kaposi sarcoma in immunodeficient patients may suggest a viral origin for this particular sarcoma [8−11].

A well-known physical agent for the development of various types of soft tissue sarcomas is ionising irradiation as employed in the therapy for other tumors [12−14]. Especially in children treated for cancer this may become a serious problem probably enhanced by genetic predisposition to multiple cancers [15]. Also long-lasting low-level irradiation from radioactive material e.g. thorothrast is implicated in the causation of Kupffer cell sarcoma in the liver [16]. Sarcomas are reported at the site of scar tissue e.g. after surgical intervention [17] and under the influence of metal implants [18].

Some chemicals are known to give rise to a particular type of soft tissue sarcoma. Angiosarcoma of the liver may develop in patients exposed to polyvinyl chloride [19, 20]. The physicochemical action of asbestos may be responsible for the development of malignant mesotheliomas [21].

Age distribution

Soft tissue sarcomas are relatively rare tumors and account for only 0.5 to 1 per cent of all malignancies. In childhood however sarcomas represent 6 to 8 per cent of all cancers [22]. Notwithstanding their rarity, soft tissue tumors constitute an important part in the field of oncology with respect to the frequent problems in diagnosis, their diverging biological behaviour and the resulting therapeutic implications. Depending on the type of sarcoma there are distinct differences in occurrence rate between the various age groups. Synovial sarcomas are neoplasms of teenagers and early adult life, whereas fibrosarcomas, liposarcomas and malignant fibrous histiocytomas are mainly seen between 40 and 60 years of age.

According to the clinical setting in which a tumor presents itself also diversities may exist in one tumor category. Haemangiosarcoma of the breast e.g. is a highly malignant lesion in young women. In elderly people a less aggressive malignant vascular neoplasm is found in the head and neck region.

Tumors occurring in childhood may be divided into two groups. Firstly the adult type tumors, meaning neoplasms more commonly seen in adults and in morphology and behaviour the same in both age groups. Secondly the typical children's tumors presumably arising froma mesenchymal blastoma and composed of an admixture of primitive mesenchymal cells and cells in various stages of differentiation. A curious fact remains that the vast majority of soft tissue sarcomas in children which display an overt malignant behaviour consist of mesenchymal cells evolving to cross-striated muscle and so have to be considered as rhabdomyosarcomas.

Diagnostic problems

Classification of malignant soft tissue tumors is often difficult. The cells of these malignant tumors often differ strongly in appearance from their tissue of origin. It is estimated that 10 to 15 per cent of soft tissue sarcomas cannot be accurately classified by routine light microscopy.

An important reason of the problems posed in diagnosis of these lesions is the relative rarity of soft tissue sarcomas coupled to a wide range of morphological varieties. So it may be very difficult for an individual pathologist, even working in a large centre, to acquire sufficient experience in this field.

Difficulties may also arise from the fact that several histological features are not unique for a given type of tumor. For example the so-called hemangiopericytomatous pattern − vessels surrounded by collars of tumor cells − is by no means specific for a hemangiopericytoma but also seen in a diverging variety of neoplasms such as leiomyosarcoma, synoviosarcoma, liposarcoma, malignant fibrohistiocytoma and myofibromatosis of infancy.

Another point is that features suggesting malignancy like cellularity, nuclear atypia, mitotic activity and infiltrative growth may be met in completely benign growths. Examples of these so-called pseudosarcomas are pleomorphic lipoma, the so-called ancient neurilemmoma and several fibromatoses of childhood.

Finally serious problems may be met in discerning soft tissue sarcomas from other categories of tumors like malignant lymphoma, undifferentiated carcinoma and melanoma. Especially pathologists, involved in childhood neoplasmas encounter difficulties in the group of the so-called small-, round-, blue-cell tumors of childhood, i.e. poorly differentiated rhabdomyosarcoma, neuroblastoma, Ewing's sarcoma and malignant non Hodgkin lymphoma [23].

A reliable morphological diagnosis is only possible on adequate material obtained by careful sampling. A cellular or structural differentiation which allows a firm diagnosis is often only present in a part of the specimen. In this respect needle biopsy or aspiration biopsy is clearly deficient. However a pathologist competent in this field of cytology may provide the clinician with a diagnosis of sarcoma with a tentative indication about type and grade which may be relevant for further intervention. Cytology is certainly useful in previously diagnosed recurrent or metastatic lesions.

Classification

In this chapter only the more common and well defined entities will be described. As indicated beforehand the relative frequency of the different types of soft tissue sarcomas depends a.o. on the age distribution of the patients. Also the criteria used to categorize these malignancies may differ. It has to be remarked that these criteria have evolved considerably during the last decades. New insights in histogenesis have profoundly altered the typing of these neoplasms. Fibrosarcoma, the most frequent sarcoma in older studies, has lost its prominent place. In recent surveys the most common soft tissue sarcomas are the malignant fibrous histiocytomas, liposarcomas, and myosarcomas followed by synoviosarcomas, angiosarcomas and fibrosarcomas.

The types of sarcoma discussed in this chapter are:
1) Malignant fibrous histiocytoma (MFH)
2) Fibrosarcoma
3) Liposarcoma
4) Leiomyosarcoma
5) Rhabdomyosarcoma
6) Vascular sarcomas
7) Malignant schwannoma
8) Synoviosarcoma
9) Chondro- and osteosarcoma of the soft parts
10) Alveolar soft part sarcoma
11) Epithelioid sarcoma
12) Clear cell sarcoma
13) Ewing sarcoma

Malignant fibrous histiocytoma (MFH)

The concept of soft tissue tumors composed of histiocytes or a combination of histiocytes and fibrocytes was reported as early as 1961 [24]. At that time a group of benign lesions was described by Kauffman and Stout under the heading of histiocytic tumors (fibrous xanthoma and histiocytoma). The malignant counter-

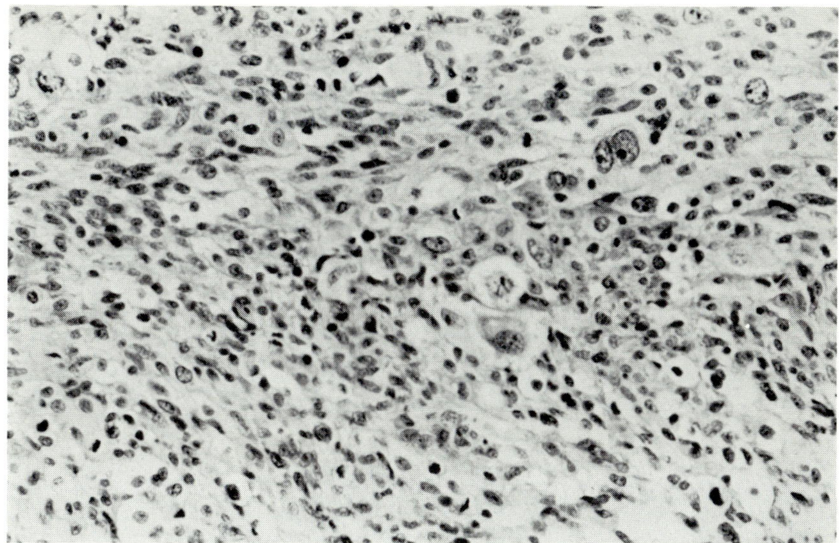

Figure 1. Malignant fibrous histiocytoma. In addition to fibroblastic differentiation, histiocyte-like tumor cells are readily found.

part was described in 1964 as malignant fibrous xanthoma [25]. These tumours were thought to arise from tissue histiocytes which could behave as 'facultative fibroblasts'. This view was supported by tissue culture studies [26] and later on by electron microscopic studies [27, 28]. The presence of proteolytic enzymes in the cells on morphologic grounds interpreted as histiocytes supported their histiocytic differentiation. The modern insights regarding the derivation of the histiocytes from precursors in the bone marrow (the monocyte-macrophage system) was difficult to reconcile with the supposed histogenesis of these soft tissue tumors. Malignancies of bone marrow derived histiocytes were delineated by modern immunochemical means and appeared to belong to a quite different nosological entity.

Recent multidisciplinary research lead to the conclusion that mesenchymal cells may differentiate into fibroblastic and histiocyte-like cells, which are encountered in this type of tumor [29]. In this sense it is understandable that during the growing acceptance of this entity the majority of formerly fibrosarcomas are labelled as MFH nowadays. A better knowledge regarding the variability of these fibrohistiocytic cells allowed to bring under this heading a number of tumors loosely attributed to pleomorphic lipo- or rhabdomyosarcomas. The 'malignant giant cell tumor of soft parts' [30, 31], formerly difficult to interpret on histogenetic grounds can now be interpreted as MFH with one-sided hystiocytic differentiation.

MFH occurs most frequently on the extremities and the retroperitoneum. Ac-

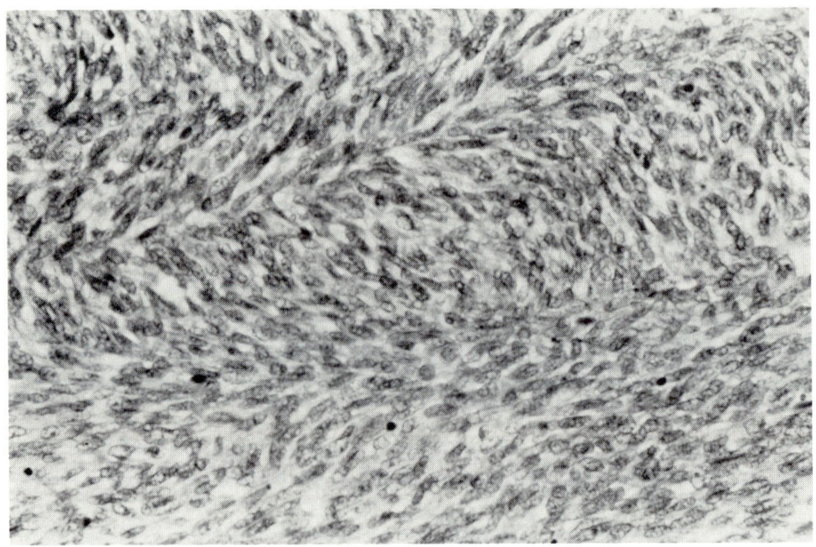

Figure 2. Fibrosarcoma. The fibroblasts are arranged in interlacing fascicles, giving rise to the so-called 'herring-bone' pattern.

cording to Enzinger and Weiss [32] they are subdivided into the following types.
1) Storiform pleomorphic
2) Myxoid
3) Giant cell
4) Inflammatory
5) Angiomatoid

The storiform-pleomorphic type consists of an intermingling of fibroblast- and histiocyte-like cells, in which particularly the last ones may exhibit a high degree of pleomorphism (Fig. 1).

Storiform relates to a configuration of especially the fibroblastic cells in which they seem to radiate from a common centre in slightly curved lines.

The myxoid type [33] is characterized by prominent myxoid change of the stroma. The giant cell type consists of numerous osteoclast-like giant cells. The inflammatory type [34] is characterized by a predominance of xanthoma cells and inflammatory cells. The angiomatoid type [35] is composed of rather uniform histiocytes with irregular blood-filled cystic spaces.

MFH is most commonly encountered in middle aged and elderly patients, except the angiomatoid type which is generally seen in patients younger than 20 years of age.

Enzinger and Weiss [32] report a metastatic rate between 40−50% for the storiform pleomorphic and giant cell type, approximately 30% for the inflammatory type and roughly 20% for the myxoid and angiomatoid type.

Fibrosarcoma

The number of cases diagnosed as fibrosarcoma has not only diminished by the acceptance of the concept of MFH but also by the recognition of fibroblastic tumors with only local agressive behaviour but without metastatic potential. Nowadays these lesions are commonly designated as agressive fibromatosis. There still remains however a place for fibrosarcomas indicating malignant tumors solely composed of fibroblast-like cells often arranged in a typical herring bone pattern (Fig. 2).

The age incidence is generally somewhat lower than for MFH. These tumors may arise in widely different places but most commonly they are seen in the extremities and on the trunk. Because of the changing diagnostic criteria it is difficult to provide a reliable survival rate from literature. In recent studies the 5 years survival ranges between 40 and 50%. It has to be kept in mind, however, that metastases may appear after the 5 years period [32].

In children is known as infantile fibrosarcoma a cellular, collagen poor neoplasm composed of undifferentiated mesenchymal cells and fibroblasts. The sites of predilection are the distal extremities. The patients are usually under the age of two, and half of the cases are congenital. The recurrence rate is 10 per cent and in 6 to 7 per cent of the cases metastases will appear [36, 37]. Infantile fibrosarcomas pursue a less aggressive clinical course than their adult counterparts.

Liposarcoma

Liposarcoma is characterized by the presence of lipoblasts. These cells contain one or more vacuoles filled with lipid material and hyperchromatic nuclei displaced to one side of the cell. In this way typical signet cell lipoblasts can be formed. With increasing lipid deposition these cells begin to approach the cellular picture of the mature fat cell.

Liposarcomas can be encountered on the extremities, trunk and head. The most frequent sites are the thigh, inguinal region and the retroperitoneum.

Liposarcomas vary considerably in their histopathological presentation and clinical behaviour. Enzinger & Weiss [32] divide liposarcomas into 4 basic histological categories i.e.
1) Well differentiated
2) Myxoid
3) Round cell
4) Pleomorphic
The well differentiated liposarcoma is characterized by the presence of mature lipocytes together with lipoblasts. Atypical cells with hyperchromatic nuclei are seen.

The myxoid liposarcoma shows a marked myxoid alteration of the stroma and

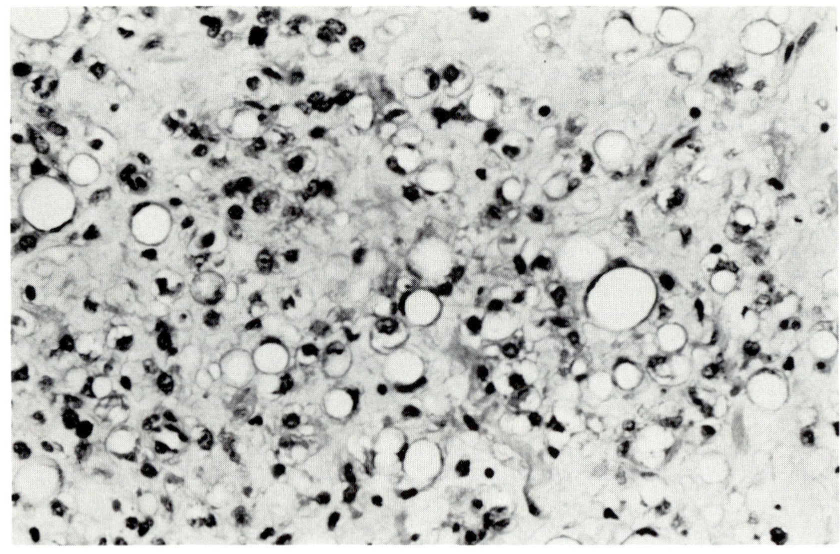

Figure 3. Myxoid liposarcoma with a myxoid matrix and lipoblasts of the 'signet-ring' type.

a peculiar plexiform network of capillaries. In addition lipoblasts are seen, mostly of the small signet ring cell type (Fig. 3).

The round cell liposarcoma is a very cellular tumor, consisting of rather uniformly shaped, rounded cells. They contain generally only a small amount of lipid material.

The pleomorphic liposarcoma is composed of large very irregular often multinucleated lipoblasts.

The recurrence rate of liposarcomas is high because these tumors tend to infiltrate over large distances, often beyond expectation. For this reason complete resection may be very difficult if not impossible. The retroperitoneal location is notorious in this respect [38, 39].

Metastases of well differentiated liposarcomas are very rare. It has to be remarked however that sometimes in well differentiated liposarcoma dedifferentiated parts are present, which may readily may give rise to metatastases. Round cell and pleomorphic liposarcoma have a high rate of metastases, up to 86% according to Enterline et al. [40]. Myxoid liposarcoma tends to have a definite lower tendency to metastasize. Especially myxoid liposarcoma may give rise to secondaries at unusual sites, often in other soft tissues. Enzinger & Weiss [32] report in almost 10% of the their patients with a primary liposarcoma of the thigh second lesions in the retroperitoneum.

Metastasizing lipomatous tumours are exceedingly rare in children. Many neoplasms diagnosed as such appear to be lipoblastomas, a benign tumor composed of lipoblasts occurring in young children. The few papers on the subject

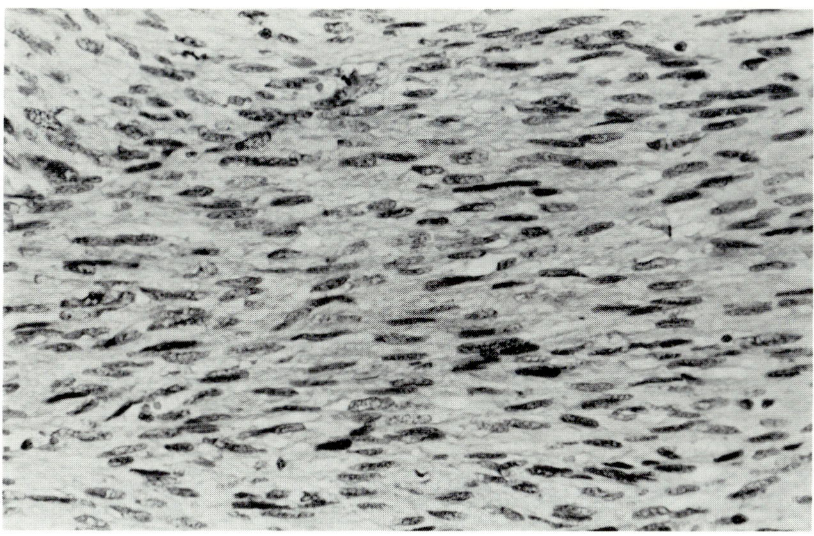

Figure 4. Well differentiated leiomyosarcoma. The tumor cells are arranged in an orderly fascicular pattern.

of liposarcomas in children report a predominance of the myxoid type and a low recurrence rate and metastatic potential [41, 42].

Leiomyosarcoma

The occurrence of leiomyosarcoma is not restricted to locations with a prominent smooth muscle component like the gastro-intestinal tract or the uterus, although in these organs smooth muscle tumours are relatively common. Outside these localisations they may be preferably encountered in the retroperitoneum the cutaneous and subcutaneous tissues. As tissue of origin smooth muscle of small vessels or along the hair follicles may be incriminated.

There is a large range of cellular differentiations in the group of leiomyosarcomas, the well differentiated sarcomas merging imperceptibly into their benign homologues, the leiomyomas. The number of mitoses is generally considered to be the most important criterium in the differentiation of the benign from the malignant smooth muscle tumors [43]. Other criteria of less importance are pleomorphism and cellularity (Figs. 4−6).

Regarding the number of mitoses a higher level seems to correlate with malignancy in the uterine tumors than e.g. in the retroperitoneal lesions. Smooth muscle tumors in the uterus with less than 5 mitoses/10 high power fields (HPF) are thought to behave as benign lesions. The prognosis for uterine leiomyosarcomas with more than 10 mitoses/10 HPF is definitely poor [44]. In retroperitoneal

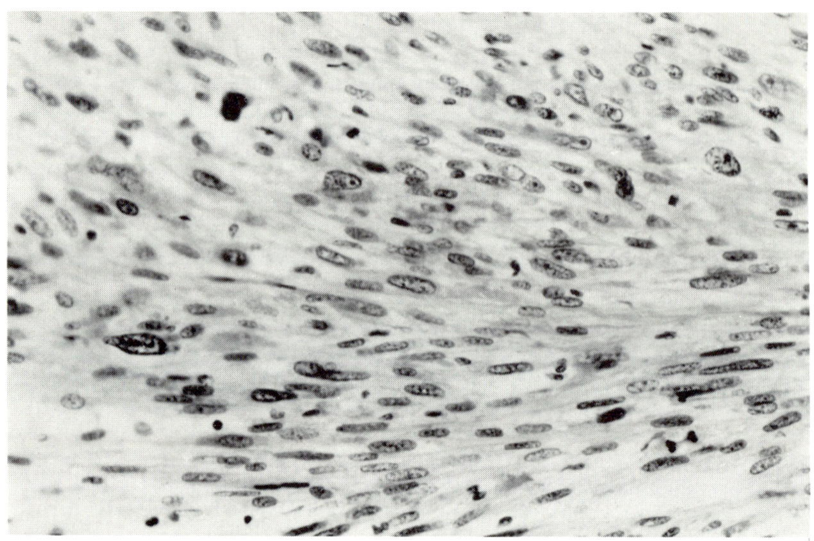

Figure 5. Moderately differentiated leiomyosarcoma. In comparison with Fig. 4. There is more pleomorphism and a greater number of mitoses. The fascicles are less orderly arranged.

smooth muscle tumors however a mitotic count between 1 and 4/10 HPF should indicate a potential malignancy and those having 5 – 9 mitoses/10 HPF have to be considered as malignant according to Enzinger and Weiss [32]. Also in gastric lesions the criteria for malignancy are difficult to assess [45]. Cutaneous and to a lesser extent subcutaneous lesions have generally a favourable prognosis. According to Fields and Helwig [46] tumors confined to the dermis do not metastasize, whereas the subcutaneous lesions metastasize in ±1/3 of the cases. Microscopically leiomyosarcomas are composed of elongated cells with more or less orderly fascicular pattern. In the less differentiated tumors, there is more pleomorphism, a higher mitotic rate and the fascicular pattern may be lost.

Sometimes the tumor cells are polygonal, rather pleomorph with a pale cytoplasm and distinct cell membranes. This 'epithelioid' differentiation is often only focally observed. Tumors, however, consisting predominantly or exclusively of these types of cells are termed leiomyoblastomas or bizarre smooth muscle tumors. They are relatively common in the gastrointestinal tract. Also in these tumors the mitotic rate is an important criterium in the differentiation between benign and malignant lesions.

Metastases of gastrointestinal leiomyosarcomas are primarily encountered in the liver and elsewhere in the abdominal cavity. Uterine leiomyosarcomas may also spread into the peritoneal cavity. Via the blood stream secondaries of the same malignancy will be found in the lungs. Metastases in lymph nodes are extremely uncommon.

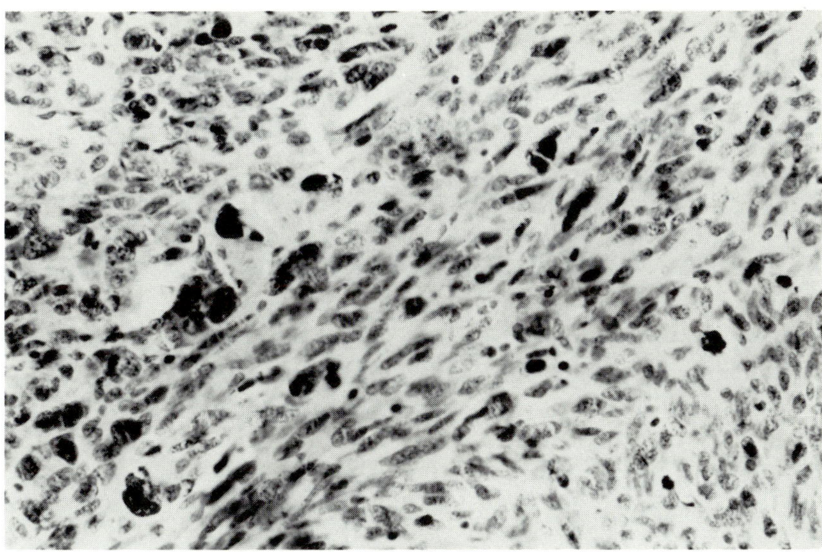

Figure 6. Poorly differentiated leiomyosarcoma. The pleomorphism is very marked. Numerous mioses are found. A fascicular pattern is hardly recognizable.

Rhabdomyosarcoma

Rhabdomyosarcomas are subdivided into three histological types, the pleomorphic (adult), the embryonal and the alveolar varieties [47]. During the last decade a remarkable shift in the occurrence rates according to age and type has taken place. In 1946, Stout [48] described pleomorphic rhabdomyosarcoma as a malignant tumor arising from the voluntary muscle in adults. As the name implies this tumor is composed of many different cell forms such as round and spindle cells, strap and raquet shaped cells and spider cells. It is realized that most cases originally reported as pleomorphic rhabdomyosarcomas are not muscle tumors at all, but pleomorphic forms of liposarcoma and malignant fibrous histiocytoma. For this reason no reliable data concerning the behaviour of this apparently exceedingly rare neoplasm are available at the moment.

In contrast stands the situation in children. In the seventies it was generally accepted that most of the soft tissue sarcomas in children consist of primitive mesenchymal cells tending to differentiate into cross-striated muscle cells and therefore defined embryonal rhabdomyosarcomas. For tumors composed only of mesenchymal cells lacking any differentiation the term embryonal sarcoma was reserved. The delineation of embryonal rhabdomyosarcoma from embryonal sarcoma is often blurred and depends a.o. on the extent of techniques used in diagnosis [49]. These embryonal tumors constitute 70 to 80% of all soft tissue sarcomas in childhood [50]. The preferred sites are the head, neck and genito-urinary region. Embryonal rhabdomyosarcomas developing from the mesenchym of mucous membranes lining cavities and hollow viscera such as vagina, bladder, biliary tree, pharynx and middle ear assume a grape-like configuration known as sarcoma botryoides. Alveolar rhabdomyosarcomas affect individuals, in an older age group, mostly in the second decade and comprise 10–15% of the rhabdomyosarcomas. This tumor shows an alveolar pattern of undifferentiated round cells and myoblasts separated by thick often hyalinized, collagenous septa. The anatomical distribution is similar to the embryonal rhabdomyosarcomas except a greater incidence in the extremities. Embryonal rhabdomyosarcomas show a tendency to remain localised and spread by direct extension with metastases confined to the regional lymphnodes. The alveolar type seems to be more aggressive and may disseminate by blood- and lymph stream early in the disease [51]. Several cases of alveolar rhabdomyosarcoma have been reported with multiple metastases from an inapparent primary [52].

An important factor with regard to prognosis is the site of the lesion. Genito-urinary and orbital tumors have a relatively good prognosis, whereas sarcomas situated in the retroperitoneal, mediastinal and parameningeal areas do badly.

With the change in treatment from surgery alone to a multidisciplinary approach survival rates have markedly improved to approximately 70 per cent [53].

Vascular tumors

Two kinds of cells typical for bloodvessels may give rise to malignant tumors i.e. endothelial cells lining blood- and lymph vessels at the inside and pericytes which are present scattered at the outside of blood capillaries.

Hemangioendotheliosarcomas or in short angiosarcomas have a predilection for the skin and superficial soft tissues in contrast to other malignant soft tissue tumors which are preferably found in the deeper soft tissues. These sarcomas are usually located in head and neck of elderly patients. They consist of irregular formed anastomosing vessels. The malignant endothelial cells may show only slight atypia, but sometimes they are markedly dedifferentiated, just reminding of rounded epithelial cells.

Clinically these tumors resemble ill-defined blue-red macules. Survival data from literature vary widely, from 30 to 75% [32]. The clinical course of vascular neoplasms in young children is, notwithstanding their cellular appearance and high mitotic activity, nearly always benign [54]. Huge lesions may be accompanied by a bleeding tendency due to platelet sequestration. A peculiar variety of hemangiosarcoma, local invasive and metastasing to the regional lymph nodes was described under the rather cumbersome name 'malignant endovascular papillary angioendothelioma of the skin' [55].

Hemangiopericytomas are vascular tumors in which the vessels are bordered by non-malignant endothelial cells. The tumor cells which fill the areas between the

− often prominent − vascular spaces are separated from the endothelial cells by delicate reticulin fibres. They are haphazardly arranged in thightly packed fields. The nuclei of these cells are generally oval and the cellular outlines are indistinct. In this type of tumor there are no reliable criteria available to predict their clinical behaviour. Increased mitotic rate − more than 4 mitoses per 10 HPF − marked pleomorphism and the presence of necrosis suggest malignant behaviour in these lesions. Haemangiopericytomas are most common in the lower extremities and in the retroperitoneum but they may be found also at other sites e.g. in the head and viscera [56]. As mentioned before, other sarcomas e.g. synoviosarcoma may have a similar vascular pattern and thereby mimick closely the histopathological picture of haemangiosarcoma.

Congenital or infantile hemangiopericytomas mostly located in the subcutaneous tissues display a benign behaviour despite histological features which would be considered ominous in older patients [56].

Malignant Schwannoma

Malignant schwannoma (synonym neurogenic sarcoma and neurofibrosarcoma) is a malignant tumor of peripheral nerves. The diagnostic criteria employed for this malignancy differ widely in literature. Some authors (Stout) adhere to a strict definition and accept only the neurogenic nature of a sarcoma if an origin from a peripheral nerve is documented or the tumor develops in a patient with Von Recklinghausen's disease. Von Recklinghausen's disease predisposes highly to this malignancy as ±10% of the patients with this disease develop a malignant schwannoma in course of time (3). Others (Enzinger) accept the diagnosis of malignant Schwannoma on histopathological grounds. According to this author, the presence of a number of rather delicate microscopic features in a fibrosarcoma-like tumor warrant the diagnosis of malignant schwannoma. These features include a.o. certain cellular irregularities, whorled arrangements of the spindle cells and the presence of hyalin bands and nodules. Ectopic tissue is more often found in this malignant schwannoma than in other types of sarcoma [57]. These ectopic tissues are seen as islands of mature cartilage, epithelial cells forming glandular structures [58, 59] and rather well differentiated cross-striated muscle. A special name (triton tumor) [60] is employed for a neurogenic tumor with skeletal muscle differentiation. Pallisading of nuclei may be a prominent feature in a malignant schwannoma. However, pallissading is also found in other sarcomas e.g. in leiomyosarcomas. Sometimes the tumor cells of a malignant schwannoma are not spindle-like but polygonal with well defined cytoplasmic membranes, resembling epithelial cells (malignant epithelioid schwannoma) which may give rise to the erroneous diagnosis of metastatic cancer.

As may be expected from the ubiquitous distribution of nerve fibres these tumors may be found in widely different locations. The 5 years survival in the material of the Armed Forces Institute of Pathology is ±50% [32]. Sordillo et al.

14

[61] report longer five-year survival for patients with solitary malignant schwannoma (47%) than for patients whose tumors developed in association with Von Recklinghausen's disease (23%).

Synoviosarcoma

A peculiar differentiation into distinct epithelial and spindle cell components is characteristic for synoviosarcoma. The epithelial cells of this neoplasm bear some resemblance to synovial cells. This feature, together with its frequent location in the vicinity of large joints suggests an origin from synovial tissues although this has never been fully substantiated. Recent studies with the aid of marker techniques have seriously challanged this conception [62].

Sometimes the epithelial but more often the spindle cell component predominates. If one of the components is hardly identifiable or absent, the designation 'monophasic' is used in contrast with the biphasic type in which both elements are obviously present (Fig. 7). It is a matter of dispute if tumors only consisting of spindle cells or − more exceptionally − only consisting of epithelial cells reliably can be diagnosed as synoviosarcoma. In order to maintain reproducible diagnostics some − even vague − biphasic pattern has to be present in our opinion or other obvious features have to sustain the diagnosis. A slight epithelial configuration can be rendered visible by the use of reticulin stains [63]. Electron microscopy may reveal characteristic structures and immunochemistry may be of considerable help in this respect (vide infra).

Synoviosarcoma is most prevalent in the younger age groups. The peak incidence is between 15 − 35 years. As mentioned beforehand, the most common location is the neighbourhood of the large joints especially of the lower limb. However, also other sites are reported e.g. the head and neck region and abdominal wall [64, 65]. A peculiar feature is the presence of multiple small foci of calcification or bone formation which can be recognized by radiologic examination.

Synoviosarcoma has to be considered as a high grade malignancy especially the poorly differentiated variant. Enzinger & Weiss [32] reports a 5-year survival rate of 45% and 16% at 10 years. The drop of the survival rate after 5 years reflects the rather frequent occurrence of late metastases.

Cartilageous and osseous tumors of the soft parts

These tumors, relatively frequent in the bony tissues are rare in the soft parts. The chondrosarcomas are found in two variants, the extraskeletal myxoid chondrosarcoma [66], as the name implies with extensive myxoid alterations of the stroma and the mesenchymal chondrosarcoma [67]. The myxoid chondrosarcoma is a slow growing tumor with a rather low potential to metastasize. Mesenchymal

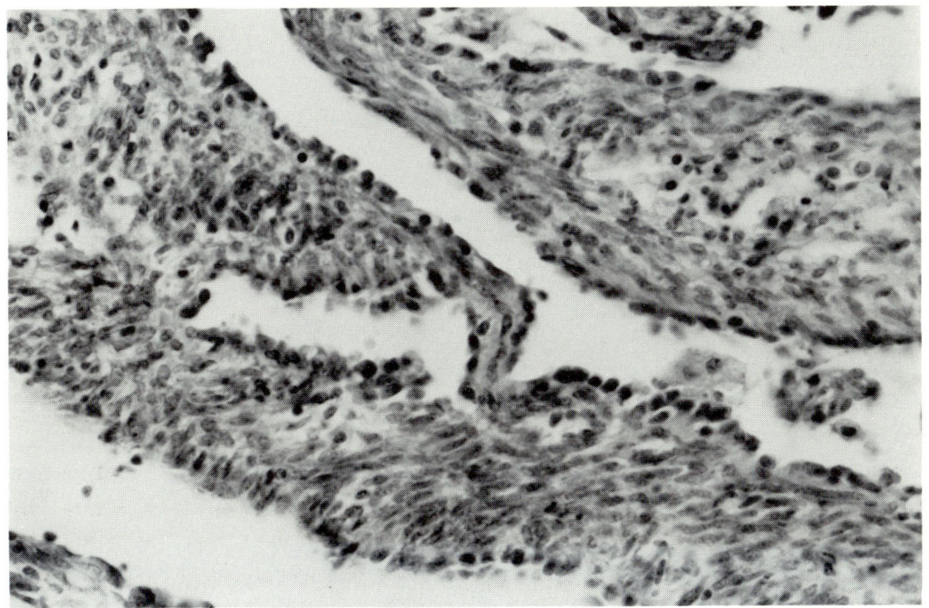

Figure 7. Synoviosarcoma with typical biphasic pattern. Cuboidal cells, lining cleft-like spaces, are surrounded by tumor cells showing fibroblastic differentiation.

chondrosarcoma, characterized by undifferentiated mesenchymal cell and islands of rather well differentiated cartilage is a very malignant tumor with a high rate of metastases. The same holds true for the osteosarcomas of the soft parts.

Sarcomas of unknown histogenesis

Some malignant soft tissue sarcomas exhibit a typical histopathological picture but do not resemble a known body structure. The histogenesis of these tumors is still a matter of dispute. To this group belong the alveolar soft part sarcoma, epithelioid sarcoma, clear cell sarcoma and Ewing sarcoma.

Alveolar soft part sarcoma

This tumor is composed of rather large cells with eosinophilic granular cytoplasm. In the cytoplasm typical crystals are observed.

The tumorcells are arranged in rather compact nests separated by delicate vessels. This is a slow growing but early metastasizing tumor, most commonly occurring in adolescents and young adults between 15−35 years of age. Sites of predilection are the lower extremities. This tumor may occur in children and in these patients it is often located in the region of head or neck.

A 5-year survival rate of 59% is reported in the literature and 20 year survival of 47% [32].

Epithelioid sarcoma

As the name implies the tumor cells of this malignancy have an epithelioid appearance. They are arranged in nodules with a typical central necrosis. It is understandable that this tumor may easily give rise to the wrong diagnosis of a metastatic cancer or even a granulomatous inflammation.

The principal sites of the neoplasm are the fingers, hands and forearms where it is found in the subcutis and deeper tissues. It has a prevalence for young adults [68]. In a large series of the AFIP [32] 76% developed one or more recurrences. Metastases occurred in 47% of the patients, most commonly in the regional lymph nodes and the lungs.

Clear cell sarcoma

The tumor cells of the clear cell sarcoma are arranged in nests or fascicles separated by fibrous septa. These cells are mostly polygonal with clear or pale cytoplasm. In ±50% of the tumor cells the presence of melanin can be demonstrated. In this connection also the term malignant melanoma of the soft parts is used to denote this tumor.

Also in clear cell sarcoma young adults are mainly afflicted. The sites of predilection are the extremities especially the region of the foot and ankle. The neoplasm is usually deep seated often connected with tendons or aponeuroses. The recurrence and metastatic rates are relatively high. In roughly 50% the tumor metastasizes, mainly to the regional lymph nodes and lungs [32].

Ewing sarcoma

During the last decade about 40 cases of a round cell soft tissue tumor were described by light microscopy and at the ultrastructural level indistinguishable from Ewing's sarcoma of bone [69, 70]. Eighty per cent occurs before the age of 30. The sites of preference are the paravertebral and intercostal regions and the lower extremities. Hematogenous metastases develop rapidly after diagnosis.

Additional techniques

Electron microscopy

The results of electron microscopy in tumor diagnosis are sometimes disappointing. A reason can be the quality of the material. Immediate and proper fixation of the tissue is a prerequisite to preserve ultrastructural detail.

Another reason is the sampling error. As a rule only groups of cells are examined by the electron microscopist which may not be representative for the lesion e.g. non neoplastic stroma cells, degenerated cell forms or cells lacking any characteristic features.

Also important to note is that relatively few cellular organelles or cell inclusions are unique for a given type of tumor. Especially for soft tissue sarcomas it holds true that at the ultrastructural level many sarcomas are composed of cells that possess basic mesenchymal features without specific characteristics. So a precise diagnosis based on electron microscopy alone is often not possible. A further difficulty pertaining to electron microscopy of soft tissue tumors is, that because of the small area examined, the architectural organisation so important in diagnosing these tumors is missing. Therefore correlation of light and electron microscopic findings remains mandatory.

Keeping the above mentioned restrictions in mind electron microscopy is extremely useful in discerning soft tissue sarcomas from other tumor categories, such as the well known differentiating problems between superficially located malignant fibrous histiocytoma and sarcomatoid skin carcinoma [71], undifferentiated round cell sarcoma and malignant lymphoma and between spindle cell sarcoma and desmoplastic amelanotic melanoma.

In the field of soft tissue growth application of electron microscopy can be especially helpful in the groups of spindle cell and round cell sarcomas. Arrays of thin filaments with densities are pathognomic for a smooth muscle origin (Figs. 8 & 9). Features suggesting a synovial tumor are microvilli lined lumina and lack of collagen production [72]. Fibrosarcomas possess a prominent rough endoplasmatic reticulum and a richly collagenous stroma. In malignant schwannoma the formation of basal membranes and the presence of slender cytoplasmic processes may be of help in diagnosis. The presence in round cell tumors of alternating thick and thin − myosin and actin − filaments and Z band material establishes the diagnosis rhabdomyosarcoma. Neurotubuli and neurosecretory granules are specific features in neuroblastoma. Cells poor in organelles, with occasionally desmosomes and rich in glycogen are suggestive for Ewing's sarcoma. However it has to be kept in mind that the undifferentiated round cells from an alveolar rhabdomyosarcoma remain also at the ultrastructural level indistinguishable from Ewing's sarcoma.

Sometimes in undifferentiated, pleomorphic tumors electron microscopy may

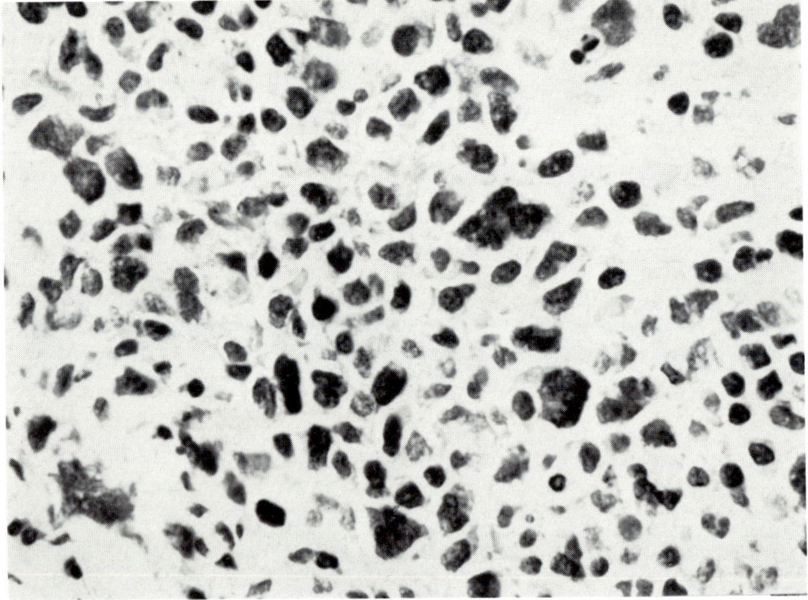

Figure 8. Female patient 65 years old. Abdominal tumors with a primary malignancy probably in the uterus. Pleomorphous malignant tumor which does not allow a classifying diagnosis (E & H stain).

be of some help (Figs. 8 & 9). Application of special stains and immuno-histochemistry will be necessary to complete the diagnosis in these cases.

A good review of the electron microscopic possibilities in soft tissue pathology is given by Henderson & Papadimitriou [73].

Special stains and markers

Already for a long time special stains are used to demonstrate various tissue elements, which can be of help to the diagnosis of soft tissue tumors. These stains are developed purely emperically and are based on often poorly understood physicochemical bands. Examples of this category are silver stains for the demonstration of reticulin fibres, van Gieson for collagen, Alcian blue for mucoid substances [74] and a variety of stains for lipid material. Later-on organic molecules or parts of molecules could be visualized by well defined histochemical reactions e.g. the PAS reaction for polysaccharides and the Feulgen reaction for DNA.

In recent years the use of (enzyme- or immune-) histochemical methods has greatly enhanced the accuracy of the morphological diagnoses of neoplasms. Enzymes can be visualized by the products of their specific activity. Complex organic

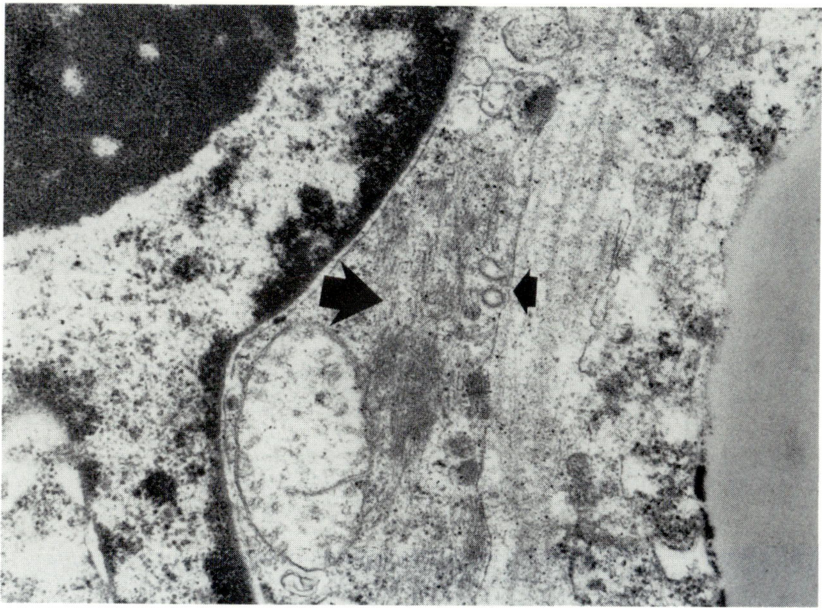

Figure 9. Same patient. On electron microscopic examination bundles of thin filaments with densities (heavy arrow) and pinocytotic vesicles (small arrow) are seen, allowing the diagnosis of leiomyosarcoma (magnif. 31.700×).

molecules, generally of proteineous nature can be pin-pointed by immunological methods.

In this respect the immunological demonstration of different types of intermediate filaments belonging to the cytoskeleton has to be mentioned. Five types of these filaments can be recognized, each of which is specific for a certain tissue type [75]. These are:

1) Cytokeratins specific for epithelial tissues
2) Vimentin found in tissues of mesenchymal origin
3) Desmin characteristic for myogenic tissues
4) The neurofilament protein, specific for neuronal tissue
5) Glial fibrillary acidic protein (GFAP), found in glial cells.

Generally these intermediate filament proteins are retained in a cell upon neoplasia. In this way carcinomas can be recognized by antibodies against (cyto) keratins in frozen sections and often also in paraffin embedded tissues. There are however exceptions. Some cancers may express both cytokeratins and vimentin (renal cell tumors, pleomorphic adenomas of salivary and sweat glands, metastatic tumor cells in pleural fluids and ascites). The same holds true for some sarcomas (vide infra).

Lymphomas generally express vimentin as do melanomas and germinomas.

Lymphomas may be recognized by a common leucocyte antibody.

Some other markers can also be of help to the diagnostics of soft tissue sarcomas. The S-100 antigen is directed against a group of acidic calcium binding proteins. It was originally isolated from brain tissue and was at that time supposed to be brain-tissue specific. Later on it became apparent that a variety of cell types and tumors express this antigen [76]. Within the group of soft tissue tumors schwannomas, granular cell tumors and tumors of cartilage are positive for S-100 antigen. Liposarcomas have been stained to show variable results whereas neuroblastomas remain unstained.

Factor VIII related antigen (antihemophilic factor) seems to be restricted to megakaryocytes, platelets and endothelial cells. The Ulex Europaeus I lectin (UEAI) binds also to endothelial cells.

The use of markers in the classification of soft tissue sarcomas

It can be helpful to apply desmin to distinguish fibrohistiocytic tumors from rhabdo- or leiomyosarcomas (Figs. 10 & 11) or S-100 antigen to distinguish them from malignant schwannomas. It has to be mentioned however that the demonstration of desmin in paraffin sections in the case of leiomyo sarcomas is variable, whereas S-100 antigens are not always detectable in malignant schwannomas. Besides desmin smooth muscle myosin is a useful marker for leiomyosarcoma.

A rather large number of markers has been described for rhabdomyosarcomas. Of these only myoglobin, skeletal muscle myosin and skeletal muscle actin have found to be specific markers for the detection of cross-striated muscle cell differentiation in tumors. Although creatin kinase subunit M and desmin are not specific for cross-striated muscle differentiation, they are very useful in distinguishing poorly differentiated rhabdomyosarcomas from other types of small round cell tumors in children.

There are no specific markers for liposarcomas. Lipid staining on frozen sections has only a very limited value, because several other tumor cells may contain also lipid material in their cytoplasm.

Factor VIII related antigen has been found in tumor cells of blood vessel endothelium, but not at all in tumor cells of haemangiopericytomas. UEAI was found to be a more sensitive marker for endothelial neoplasms.

Of practical importance is the coexpression for cytokeratin and vimentin in a number of soft tissue sarcomas. Whereas the epithelial cells of synoviosarcomas contain keratin, the spindle cells of these tumors are decorated by vimentin and keratin. The same is found in the tumor cells of epithelioid sarcomas. This feature may be of help to distinguish epithelioid sarcoma from malignant melanoma, necrotising granuloma and MFH. Antibodies against neurofilaments have been shown to be of little value in the diagnosis of neuroblastoma. Neurofilaments can usually only be detected in ganglion-like cells and in some highly differentiated

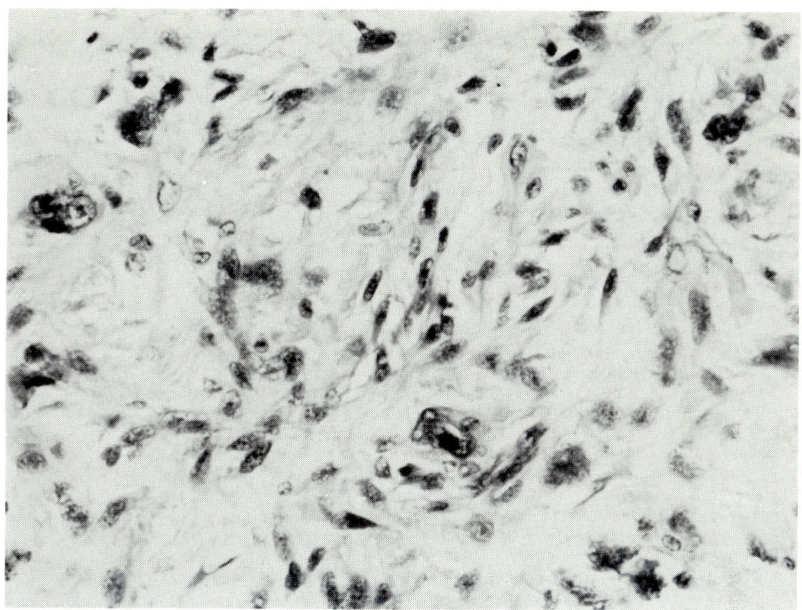

Figure 10. Large tumor on the thoracic wall in a female patient 40 years old. Light microscopically the diagnosis MFH was made.

forms of neuroblastoma. Roholl et al. [77] report that poorly differentiated neuroblastomas do not stain for any type of intermediate filament proteins. Ewing's sarcoma, rhabdomyosarcoma or lymphoma which can be difficult to differentiate from neuroblastoma on morphologic grounds stain in all cases with an antibody to vimentin when frozen sections are used. Therefore a negative reaction with all intermediate filament antibodies is an indication of neuroblastoma.

From the foregoing it is clear that these markers can be a useful tool in the diagnosis of soft tissue sarcomas. It has to be emphasized however that it never replaces the histopathological observation. Careful sampling and histomorphology still provide the most important criteria for the diagnosis of neoplasms.

Grading of soft tissue sarcomas

It is apparent that some types of soft tissue sarcomas have a very poor prognosis e.g. rhabdomyosarcoma, neuroblastoma. They have to be considered as high grade malignancies [78]. Other sarcomas can be subdivided into variants with different clinical behaviour. A good example of the last category are the liposarcomas as described beforehand [79]. The well differentiated liposarcoma practically does not metastasize, the round cell and in particular the pleomorphic liposarcomas are high grade tumors which metastasize in a high percentage.

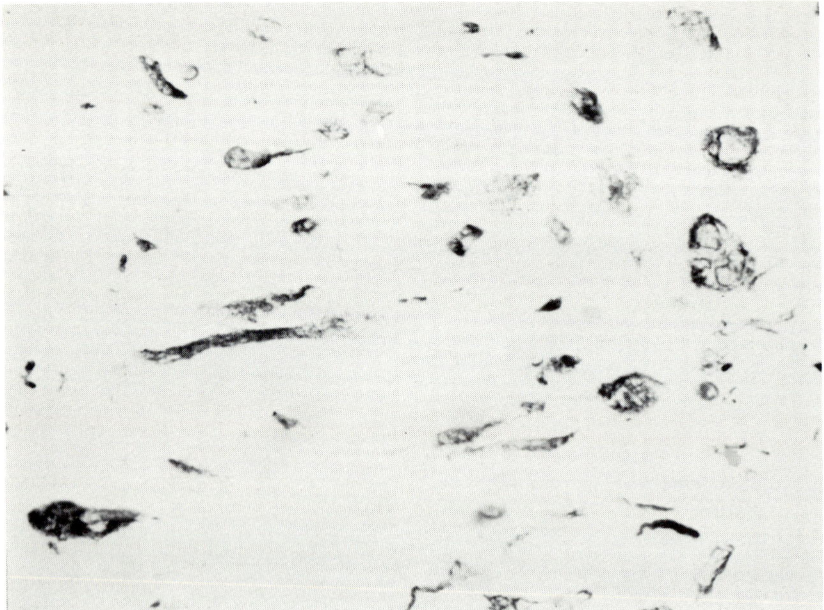

Figure 11. Desmin was clearly positive in the cytoplasm of the tumor cells in accordance with a leiomyosarcoma. The diagnosis leiomyosarcoma was confirmed electron microscopically. The smooth muscle differentiation was also light microscopically more clearly expressed after growth of a tumor implantation in a nude mouse.

In the fibrocytic tumors, the variant with only local agressiveness and without the capability to metastasize, is a well recognisable entity and by its name separated from the sarcomas i.e. aggressive fibromatosis. There remain however some relative frequent types of soft tissue sarcomas which exhibit a large range in clinical behaviour, namely the group of fibrohistiocytic sarcomas, the leiomyosarcomas and the malignant schwannomas. In this group there is a definite need for a reliable grading system. Moreover in subtypes such as the myxoid liposarcomas and in some other tumortypes (e.g. vascular tumors) it is worthwhile to investigate the possibility to recognize the cases with lower and higher potential to metastasize.

From the data in literature many features appear to be correlated with prognosis e.g. cellularity, pleomorphisms, the amount of myxoid or fibrillar matrix, mitotic rate and necrosis [80]. There is a growing consensus that mitotic rate and necrosis are the most important denominators in this respect [81–84]. Trojani et al. [84] attach a certain value to the grades in which the relevant histopathological features are represented. They use e.g. the numbers 1 to 3 related to degrees of differentiation or the number of mitoses assembled into three groups. By making an addition of the values obtained they arrive at a 'score' which is related to a certain degree of malignancy. In this way their cases of sarcomas are divided into

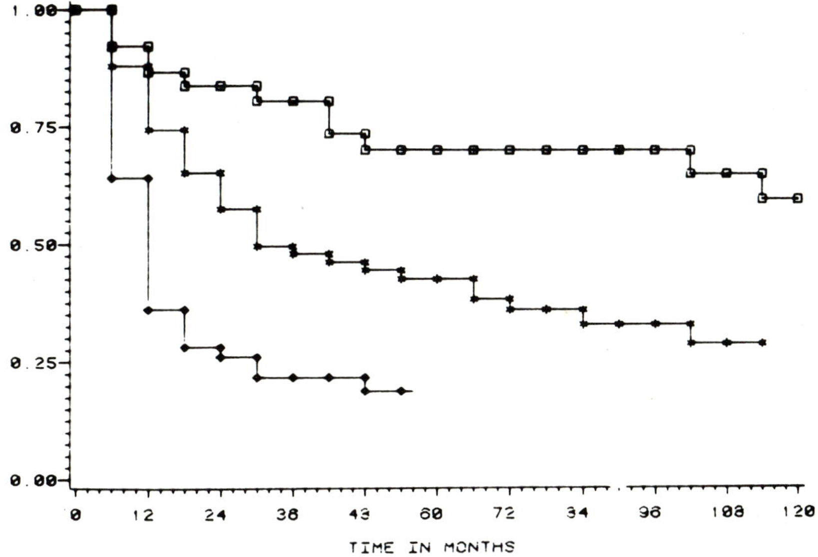

Figure 12. Survival curves according to tumor grade □ Grade 1, 39 patients, *, grade 2, 66 patients, ◇ grade 3, 50.

3 grades apparently related to survival (Fig. 12). It has to be seen which method gives the most relevant and reproducible information for there is a definite need for a uniform grading system.

Soft tissue tumors are notoriously heterogeneous. Consequently adequate sampling is of prime importance for reliable typing and grading.

Finally it has to be emphasized that the division in grades of malignancy is a simplification. The clinical behaviour of soft tissue sarcomas is more complex than can be derived from a grading system. For the decision to administer cytostatics as adjuvant therapy it is indispensable to have insight in the chance of metastases of a given tumor. A slow growing but easily metastasizing sarcoma may be a candidate for adjuvant therapy but to evaluate the results, a long follow up is necessary.

References

1. Enneking W. F., Spanier S. S., Goodman M. A. (1980) A system for the surgical staging of musculoskeletal sarcoma. Clin. Orthop. & Rel. Res. 153: 106 – 120.
2. Enzinger F. M., Lattes R., Torloni R. (1969). Histological typing of soft tissue tumours. International Classification of tumours no. 3. World Health Organization. Geneva.
3. D'Agostino A. N., Soule E. H., Miller R. H. (1963) Sarcomas of the peripheral nerves and so-

matic soft tissues associated with multiple neurofibromatosis. Cancer 16: 1015 – 1027.

4. Birch J. M., Hartley A. L., Marsden H. B., Harris M. and Swindell R. (1984) Excess Risk of Breast Cancer in the Mothers of Children with Soft Tissue Sarcomas. Br. J. Cancer 49: 325 – 331.

5. Li F. P. and Fraumeni J. F. Jr. (1969) Soft tissue Sarcomas, Breast Cancer and other Neoplasms. A familial Syndrome? Ann. Int. Med. 71: 747 – 752.

6. McKeen E. A., Bodurtha J., Meadows A. T., Douglass E. C. and Mulvihill J. J. (1978) Rhabdomyosarcoma complicating Multiple Neurofibromatosis. J. Pediatr. 94: 173 – 174.

7. Schweisguth O., Gerard-Marchant R. and Lemerle J. (1968) Naevomatose Baso-Cellulare: Association à un Rhabdomyosarcome congenital. Arch. Franc. Pédiat. 25: 1083 – 1093.

8. Abrams D. I. (1984) Hematologic manifestations in homosexual men with Kaposi's sarcoma. Am. J. Clin. Path. 81: 13 – 18.

9. Akhtar M, Bunuan H., Ashraf M., Godwin J. T. (1984) Kaposi's sarcoma in renal transplant recipients. Cancer 53: 258 – 263.

10. Boldogh I., Beth E., Huang E. S., Kyalwazi S. K., Giraldo G. (1981) Kaposi sarcoma, detection of CMV (cytomegalovirus) DNA, CMV-RNA and CMV determined nuclear antigen(s) in tumor biopsies. Int. J. Cancer 28: 469 – 474.

11. Ueda G. (1984) Kaposi's sarcoma and angioimmunoblastic lymphadenopathy. Cancer 54: 1582 – 1586.

12. Alpert L. I. (1973) Radiation induced extraskeletal osteosarcoma. Cancer 31: 1359 – 1363.

13. Davies J. D., Rees, G. J. G., Mera S. L. (1983) Angiosarcoma in irradiated postmastectomy chest wall. Histopathol. 7: 947 – 956.

14. Halpern J., Kapolovic J., Catane R. (1984) Malignant fibrous histiocytoma developing in irradiated sacral chordoma. Cancer 53: 2661 – 2662.

15. Miké V., Meadows A. T. and D'Angio G. J. (1982) Incidence of second malignant Neoplasms in Children: Results of an International Study. Lancet 2: 1326 – 1331.

16. Falk H., Telles N. C., Ishak K. G., Thomas L. B., Popper H. (1979) Epidemiology of thorotrast induced hepatic angiosarcoma in the United States. Environ. Res. 18: 65 – 73.

17. Inoshita T. (1984) MFH arising in previous surgical sites. Cancer 53: 176 – 183.

18. Lee Y. S., Pho R. W. H., Nather A. (1984) Malignant fibrous histiocytoma at the site of a metal implant. Cancer 54: 2286 – 2290.

19. Evans D. M., Jones Williams W., Kung I. T. (1983) Angiosarcoma and hepatocellular carcinoma in vinyl chloride workers. Histopathol. 7: 377 – 388.

20. Thomas L. B., Popper H. (1975) Pathology of angiosarcoma of the liver among vinyl chloride polyvinyl chloride workers. Annals N. York Acad. of Science 246: 268 – 277.

21. Belleau R., Gaensler E. A. (1968) Mesothelioma and asbestos. Respirations 25: 67 – 79.

22. Birch J. M., Marsden H. B. and Swindell R. (1980) Incidence of malignant Disease in Childhood: A 24-year Review of the Manchester Children's Tumour Registry Data. Br. J. Cancer 42: 215 – 223.

23. Triche T. J., Askin F. B. (1983) Neuroblastoma and the differential diagnosis of small-, round-, blue-Cell Tumors. Hum. Pathol. 14: 569 – 595.

24. Kauffman S. L., Stout A. P. (1961) Histiocytic tumors (fibrous xanthoma and histiocytoma) in children. Cancer 14: 469 – 482.

25. O'Brien J. E., Stout A. P. (1964) Malignant fibrous xanthomas. Cancer 17: 1445 – 1455.

26. Ozzello L., Stout A. P., Murray M. R. (1963) Cultural characteristics of malignant histiocytomas and fibrous xanthomas. Cancer 16: 331 – 344.

27. Harris M. (1980) The ultrastructure of benign and malignant fibrous histiocytomas. Histopathol. 4: 29 – 44.

28. Fu Y., Gabbiani G., Kaye G. I., Lattes R. (1975) Malignant soft tissue tumors of probable histiocytic origin (Malignant fibrous histiocytomas): general considerations and electron microscopic and tissue culture studies. Cancer 35: 176 – 198.

29. Roholl P. J. M., Kleyne J., Van Basten C. D. H., Van der Putte S. C. J., Van Unnik J. A. M. (1985) A study to analyse the origin of tumor cells in malignant fibrous histiocytomas: a multiparameter characterization. Cancer 56: 2809–2815.

30. Alguacil-Garcia J., Unni K. K., Goellner J. R. (1977) Malignant giant cell tumor of soft parts. Cancer 40: 244–253.

31. Angervall L., Heymar B., Kindblom L. G., Merck C. (1981) Malignant giant cell tumor of soft tissues. Cancer 47: 736–747.

32. Enzinger F. M., Weiss S. W. (1983) Soft tissue tumors. The C. V. Mosby Company St. Louis-Toronto-London.

33. Lagace R., Delage C., Seemayer T. A. (1979) Myxoid variant of malignant fibrous histiocytoma. Cancer 43: 526–534.

34. Kyriakos M., Kempson R. L. (1976) Inflammatory fibrous histiocytoma. Cancer 37: 1584–1606.

35. Enzinger F. M. (1979) Angiomatoid malignant fibrous histiocytoma. Cancer 44: 2147–2157.

36. Chung E. B. and Enzinger F. M. (1976) Infantile Fibrosarcoma Cancer 38: 729–739.

37. Soule E. H. and Pritchard D. J. (1977) Fibrosarcoma in Infants and Children. A Review of 110 Cases. Cancer 40: 1711–1721.

38. Cody H. S., Turnbull A. D., Fortner J. G., Hajdu S. I. (1981) The continuing challenge of retroperitoneal sarcoma. Cancer 47: 2147–2152.

39. Evans H. L., Soule E. H., Winkelman R. K. (1979) Atypical lipoma, atypical intramuscular lipoma and well differentiated retroperitoneal liposarcoma. Cancer 43: 574–584.

40. Enterline H. T., Culberson J. D., Rochlin D. B., Bradly L. W. (1960). Liposarcoma – a clinical and pathological study of 53 cases. Cancer 13: 932–950.

41. Castleberry R. P., Kelly D. R., Wilson E. R., Cain W. S. and Salter M. R. (1984) Childhood Liposarcoma. Report of a Case and Review of the Literature. Cancer 54: 579–584.

42. Smookler B. M. and Enzinger F. M. (1983) Liposarcoma occurring in Children. An Analysis of 17 Cases and Review of the Literature. Cancer 52: 567–574.

43. Ranchod M., Kempson R. L. (1977) Smooth muscle tumors of the gastrointestinal tract and retroperitoneum. Cancer 39: 255–262.

44. Kempson R. L., Bari W. (1970) Uterine sarcomas: classification, diagnosis and prognosis. Human Path. 1: 331–350.

45. Morson B. C., Dawson I. M. P. (1979) Gastro-intestinal pathology. Blackwell Scientific Publications Oxford, London, Edinburgh, Melbourne p. 189.

46. Fields J. P., Helwig E. B. (1981) Leiomyosarcoma of the skin and subcutaneous tissue. Cancer 47: 156–169.

47. Horn R. C. and Enterline H. T. (1958) Rhabdomyosarcoma: A clinicopathological Study and Classification of 39 Cases. Cancer 11: 181–199.

48. Stout A. P. (1946) Rhabdomyosarcoma of the skeletal Muscle. Ann. Surg. 123: 447–472.

49. Kahn H. J., Yeger H., Kassim O., Jorgensen A. O., MacLennan D. H., Baumal R., Smith C. R. and Phillips M. J. (1983) Immunohistochemical and electron microscopic Assessment of Childhood Rhabdomyosarcoma. Increased Frequency of Diagnosis over routine histologic Methods. Cancer 51: 1897–1903.

50. Jenkin R. D. T. (1972) Rhabdomyosarcoma in Childhood. In Cancer in Childhood. Godden J. O. (ed) The Ontario Cancer Treatment and Research Foundation Toronto. 157–165.

51. D'Angio G. J. and Evans A. (1975) Soft Tissue Sarcomas. In 'Cancer in Children, Clinical Management' Bloom H. J. G., Lemerle J., Neidhardt M. K. and Voûte P. A. (ed). Springer-Verlag Berlin Heidelberg New York. 217–241.

52. Almanaseer I. Y., Trujillo Y. P., Taxy J. B. and Okuno T. (1984) Systemic Rhabdomyosarcoma with diffuse Bone Marrow Involvement. Am. J. Clin. Pathol. 82: 349–353.

53. Maurer H. M. (1979) Rhabdomyosarcoma. Pediatr. Ann. 8: 35–48.

54. Taxy J. B. and Gray S. R. (1979) Cellular Angiomas of Infancy. Cancer 43: 2322–2331.

55. Dabska M. (1969) Malignant endovascular papillary Angioendothelioma of the Skin in Childhood Cancer 24: 503 – 510.

56. Enzinger F. M. and Smith B. H. (1970) Hemangiopericytoma. An Analysis of 106 Cases. Hum.
Pathol. 7: 61 – 82.

57. Ducatman B. S., Scheithauer B. (1984) Malignant peripheral nerve sheat tumors with divergent
differentiation. Cancer 54: 1049 – 1057.

58. Uri A. K., Witzleben C. L., Ravey B. (1984) Electron microscopy of glandular schwannoma.
Cancer 53: 493 – 497.

59. Woodruff J. M. (1976) Peripheral nerve tumors showing glandular differentiation. Cancer 37:
2399 – 2413.

60. Woodruff J. M., Chernik N. L., Smith M. C., Millett W. B., Foote F. W. (1973) Peripheral
nerve tumors with rhabdomyosarcomatous differentiation (malignant 'triton' tumors). Cancer
32: 426 – 439.

61. Sordillo P. P., Helson L., Hajdu S. I., Magill G. B., Kosloff C., Golbey R. G., Beattie E. J.
(1981) Malignant Schwannoma Clinical Characteristics, Survival and Response to Therapy. Cancer 47: 2503 – 2509.

62. Virtanen I., Miettinen M. (1984) Synovial sarcoma – a misnomer. Am. J. of Pathol. 117:
18 – 25.

63. Mackenzie D. H. (1977) Monophasic synovial sarcoma, a histological entity? Histopathology 1:
151 – 157.

64. Pack G. T., Ariel I. M. (1950) Synovial sarcoma (malignant synovioma) a report of 60 cases.
Surgery 28: 1047 – 1084.

65. Hale J. E., Calder I. (1970) Synoviosarcoma of the abdominal wall. Br. J. Cancer 24: 471 – 474.

66. Enzinger F. M., Shiraki M. (1972) Extraskeletal myxoid chondrosarcoma. Human Path. 3:
421 – 441.

67. Guccion J. G., Font R. L., Enzinger F. M., Zimmerman E. (1973) Extraskeletal mesenchymal
chondrosarcoma. Arch. Pathol. 95: 336 – 340.

68. Enzinger F. M. (1970) Epithelioid sarcoma: a sarcoma simulating a granuloma or a carcinoma.
Cancer 26: 1029 – 1041.

69. Soule E. H. Newton W. Moon T. E. and Teft M. (1978) Extraskeletal Ewing's Sarcoma. A
preliminary Review of 26 Cases encountered in the Intergroup Rhabdomyosarcoma Study. Cancer 42: 259 – 264.

70. Angervall L. and Enzinger F. W. (1975) Extraskeletal Neoplasm resembling Ewing's Sarcoma.
Cancer 36: 240 – 251.

71. Harris M. (1982) Spindle cell squamous carcimona: ultrastructural observations. Histopathol. 6:
197 – 210.

72. Mickelson M. R., Brown G. A., Maynard J. A., Cooper R. R., Bonfiglio M. (1980) Synovial
sarcoma. An electron microscopic study of monophasic and biphasic forms. Cancer 45:
2109 – 2118.

73. Henderson D. W. and Papadimitriou J. M. (1982) Ultrastructural Appearances of Tumours.
Churchill Livingstone. Edinburgh London Melbourne New York, pp. 200 – 269.

74. Mackenzie D. H. (1983) The unsuspected soft tissue chondrosarcoma. Histopathol. 7: 759 – 766.

75. Ramaekers F. C. S., Puts J. J. G., Moesber O., Kant A., Huysmans A., Haag D., Jap P. H.
K., Herman C. J., Vooys G. P. (1983) Antibodies to intermediate filament proteins in the immunohistochemical identification of human tumors: an overview. Histochem. J. 15: 691 – 713.

76. Weiss S. W., Langloss J. M., Enzinger F. M. (1983) Value of S-100 protein in the diagnosis of
soft tissue tumors with particular reference to benign and malignant schwann cell tumors. Lab.
Investigation 49: 299 – 308.

77. Roholl P. J. M., De Jong A. S. H., Ramaekers F. C. S. (1985) Application of markers in the
diagnosis of soft tissue tumours. Histopathology, 9: 1019 – 1035.

78. Russell W. O., Cohen J., Enzinger F. M., Hajdu S. I., Heise H., Martin R. G., Meissner W.,

Miller W. T., Schmitz R. L., Suit H. D. (1977) A clinical and pathological staging system for soft tissue sarcomas. Cancer 40: 1562 – 1570.

79. Reitan J. B., Kaalhus O., Breunhoud I. O., Sager E. M., Stenwig A. E., Table K. (1985) Prognostic factors in liposarcoma. Cancer 55: 2482 – 2490.

80. Markhede G., Angervall L., Stener B. (1982) A multivariate analysis of the prognosis after surgical treatment of malignant soft tissue tumors. Cancer 49: 1721 – 1733.

81. Costa J., Wesley R. A., Glatstein E., Rosenberg S. A. (1984) The grading of soft tissue sarcomas. Cancer 53: 530 – 541.

82. De Stefani E., Deneo-Pellegrini H., Carzoglio J., Cendam M. E., Vassalo A., Coppola J., Olivera L., Viola A. (1982) Sarcomes des tissus mous: facteurs histologiques de pronostic. Bull Cancer 69: 443 – 450.

83. Myhre-Jensen O., Kaal S., Hjallund Madsen E., Sneppen O. (1983) Histopathological grading in soft tissue tumours. Acta Path. Microbiol. Immunol. Scand. Sect. 91: 145 – 150.

84. Trojani M., Contesso G., Coindre J. M. et al. (1984) Soft tissue sarcomas of adults: Study of pathological and prognostic variables and definition of a histological grading system. Int. J. Cancer 33: 37 – 42.

2. Diagnostic strategy for adult soft tissue sarcomas

David E. Markham

Accurate histological diagnosis, coupled with a detailed knowledge of the local extent of the tumour along with it's spread to more distant parts, is essential for the efficient overall management of soft tissue sarcomas. Whilst other methods of treatment are available for temporary control of these tumours, surgery remains the most effective method. The local extent of the tumour must be accurately determined. Imaging techniques are important in this respect and must be used before histological biopsy. Their results, in addition to being more accurate and less prone to misinterpretation before biopsy, may indicate other essential investigations which are necessary before definitive biopsy is undertaken. This chapter will detail a diagnostic strategy for the evaluation behaviour of the tumour and will include a medical history and physical examination, scintigraphy, conventional and computed imaging, arteriorgraphy and surgical biopsy.

Anatomical Characteristics of Soft Tissue Sarcomas

An understanding of the local behaviour and potential for metastatic spread of the tumours in this class is essential to their systematic diagnostic evaluation. It would seem that soft tissue sarcomas arise in a single microscopic site and grow in a centrifugal manner. Tumour cells on the periphery, along with adjacent normal tissue cells become compressed and layered by growth of the tumour, giving the appearance of encapsulation. However, this pseudo-capsule, which is composed of normal inflammatory cells, oedematous soft tissue and peripheral tumour cells, is sporadically penetrated by microscopic extensions of the tumour, resulting in small satellite colonies of malignant cells anatomically situated well outside the apparent boundaries of this pseudo-capsule. Occasionally, such a satellite colony may be found a considerable distance from the primary tumour but still probably representing extension rather than metastasis [1].

Soft tissue sarcomas are known to respect anatomical compartments in their local early growth and spread. They respect major fascial planes and remain limit-

Pinedo, H. M., Verweij, J (eds) Clinical Management of Soft Tissue Sarcomas
© *1986 Martinus Nijhoff Publishers, Boston. ISBN 0-89838-808-2. Printed in The Netherlands.*

30

ed to well defined anatomical compartments, that is compartments whose boundaries are fascia, bone or articular cartilage, until a late stage in their development or unless they are disrupted by surgical intervention. Thus it is obvious that biopsy may contaminate a second anatomical compartment, facilitating tumour spread. Tumours arising outside a well defined anatomical compartment, for example the popliteal fossa or the femoral triangle, can spread greater distances without encountering anatomical barriers.

Major nerves and vessels tend to be displaced rather than invaded. However, they do provide an anatomical pathway for tumour spread, particularly those tumours arising outside major fascial compartments.

Metastasis is usually blood born and occurs more commonly in the lungs, liver and bone [2]. Regional lymph node involvement is relatively rare but, when it does occur, is a bad prognostic sign [3]. It is, in fact, equivalent to metastatic spread.

This simplistic approach to the histological and anatomical behaviour of soft tissue sarcomas does provide a logical basis for its investigation and surgical treatment, although it does not consider the possible systemic spread of the disease.

Medical history and physical examination

The most common clinical presentation is that of a patient with a painless swelling of relatively short duration. However, there are slow growing tumours in this group and it is not uncommon to obtain a history of a swelling which has been present for some years. Patients are typically, but not exclusively, aged between twenty and sixty years. The disease equally affects both sexes.

The medical history should include questions about systemic symptoms, the general state of health, and weight loss.

Routine laboratory investigations should include a hemoglobin, full blood count, urinalysis, erythrocyte sedimentation rate and biochemistry. Whilst abnormal results of these investigations are not diagnostic, they do act as a base line when evaluating the effects of treatment.

Detailed examination of the tumour for site, size, shape, consistence, mobility, tenderness and warmth should be followed by a thorough examination of the affected area for muscle wasting, limited movement of, and effusions into, joints. An assessment of the peripheral circulation of the limb should be made. Circulation is not usually affected unless the tumour becomes very large and causes circulatory embarrassment by mechanical compression. Similarly, it is rare to find neurological complications in these patients, since the tumour tends to displace nerves rather than invade them. Regional lymph nodes should be palpated for enlargement indicating potential infiltration with malignant cells. A general examination should follow. This should include clinical examination of the chest and abdomen for possible metastatic invasion of the lung or liver. In the case of a pelvic tumour, rectal and pelvic examinations may be of some assistance in its physical assessment.

Simple Diagnostic Imaging

Radiological assessment starts with standard x-rays in two planes. They can give an indication of the anatomical site, size, and on occasions, the internal characteristics of certain tumours as, for example, ectopic calcification found within some sarcomas [4]. Unfortunately, these tumours are usually of water density making standard x-rays relatively unhelpful in their diagnosis. However, sometimes the conventional radiograph may reveal involvement of adjacent bones or neighbouring joints.

Xeroradiography is not accurate. False negatives are common, particularly when the tumour mass is isodense.

Extremity tumors are well approachable by ultrasound since they are not covered by overlying bowel gas or by thick layers of adipose tissue. Distinct separating interfaces may be found, because most soft tissue lesions have an acoustic impedance which is different from that of surrounding normal tissue. The ability to detect these differences, coupled with the opportunity to visualize the tissue in transverse and longitudinal planes yields a sonogram with a clear and accurate reproduction of the lesion. Although some argue that ultrasound is more sensitive than computed tomography in detecting small tumours, more accurate in measuring tumour extent and size, and simpler to use without exposing the patient to excessive amounts of irradiation, it is however, less accurate in demonstrating individual muscle groups and vascular structures, particularly in complex anatomical sites [5].

Complex Diagnostic Imaging

Computed axial tomography is particularly helpful in delineating the local extent of soft tissue tumours [6, 7]. It detects tissue gross distortions of the normal anatomy, and density differences between the normal muscle, fascia or bone and the tumour (Fig. 1). Injections of contrast material during the scan enhances neighbouring structures, increasing the accuracy of the image and has eliminated many of the previous false negatives which were obtained when the tumour was small, isodense or nondisruptive to the normal anatomy. This particular investigation is most useful in areas where the anatomy is complicated, such as the pelvis, the retroperitoneum, the shoulder girdle or the proximal thigh. Surgical and pathological correlation with pre-operative computed tomography shows it to be an extremely accurate investigation in determining the transverse extent of a tumour, including it's relationship to local muscles, soft tissue and bone. The longitudinal

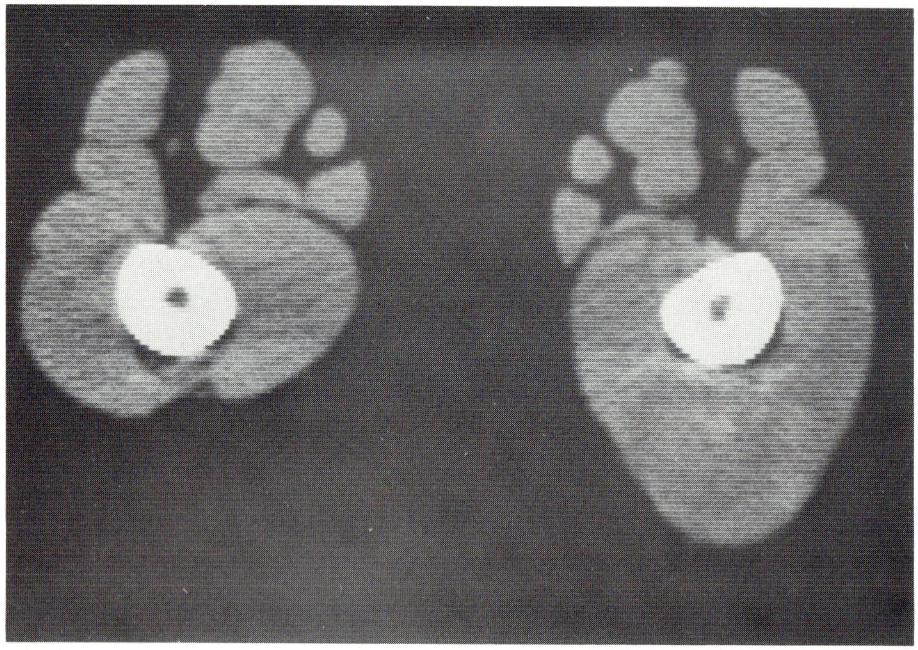

Figure 1. CT-scan of the thigh showing a lesion with different density from muscle and indicating tumor margins.

extent is not, unfortunately, so reliable, due to the difficulty of estimating the distal and proximal borders within the terminal cuts. Identification of soft tissue masses and the character of their borders, that is whether they are infiltrative or whether they represent a pseudo-capsule, is usually possible with computed tomography.

Research into, and the development of, Nuclear Magnetic Resonance suggests that this imaging technique will eventually attain the accuracy of computed axial tomography. It already has distinct advantages in the investigation of tumours arising from the nervous system, where it's accuracy is greater than that of computer tomography. However, as yet, there is no current advantage in the use of this technique for soft tissue sarcomas.

Although arteriography can not reliably distinguish between benign and malignant tumours it does have a prominent role in the pre-operative assessment of soft tissue tumours [8]. It is very effective in outlining the extra osseous extent of a tumour and is superior to any other currently available technique in outlining it's vascular anatomy, identifying the invasion of vessels, the proximity of major vessels and the site of 'feeder vessels'. This technique may yield useful information about the blood supply to, and venous drainage from, the tumour which enables the surgeon to plan his surgical attack on the tumour in such a way as to minimize tumour embolisation during surgery in addition to controlling the blood supply

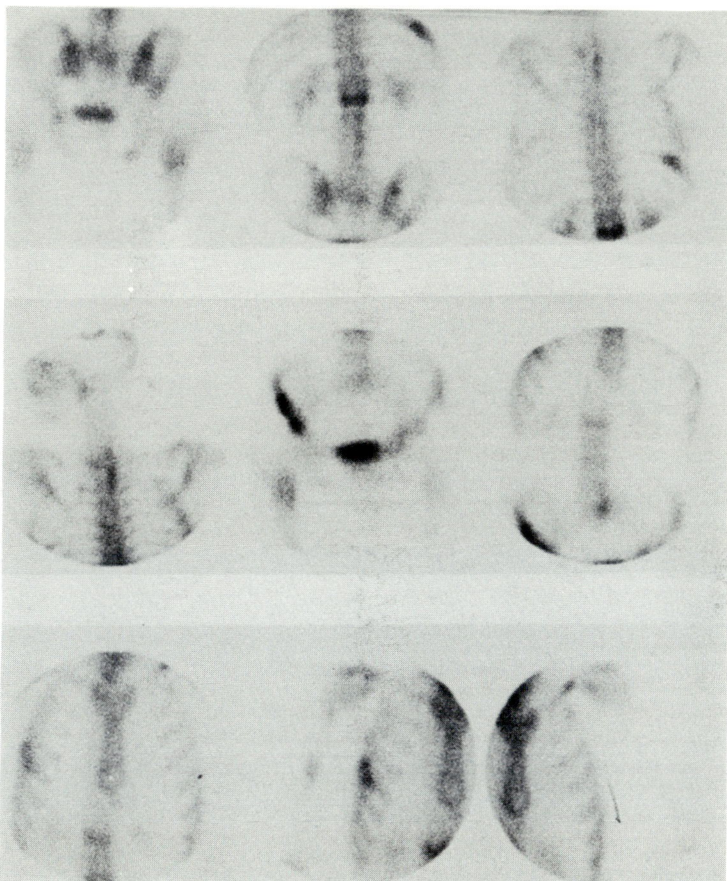

Figure 2. Details of technetium-99m phosphonate bone scan demonstrating bone metastases a synoivial sarcoma in a rib, the second lumber vertebra, the right iliac crest, the right femur, the right humerus and the skull.

to the mass. The appearance of 'blood lakes' on angiography is an indication of the aggresive nature of the tumour since they indicate rapid tumour growth. Angiography is particularly helpful in assessment of peripheral tumours. The results of this investigation are less helpful in tumours of the pelvis, trunk and shoulder girdle where computed tomography is of greater assistance.

Scintigraphic Imaging

Bone scanning using Technetium − 99m polyphosphate enjoys a dual role in the pre-operative assessment of soft tissue sarcomas. Whilst highly vascular, rapidly growing, tumours may themselves show soft tissue scintigraphic intensity, the

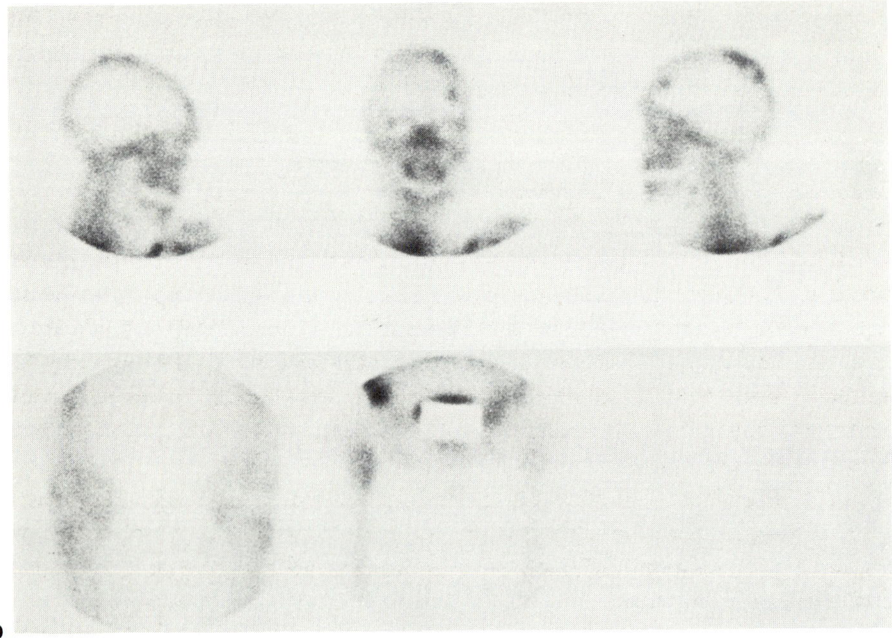

Figure 2. Continued.

main advantages of this investigation are in the staging of the primary tumour and the detection of distant bony metastases (Fig. 2).

Where increased focal intensity in bone adjacent to the primary tumour may suggest actual bone invasion by that tumour, it should be remembered that the reactive tissue zone between the lesion and bone is very narrow. Therefore that increased intensity in adjacent bone may not necessarily indicate bone invasion but does indicate proximity of the tumour to bone sufficient to affect the staging of the tumour and, therefore, it's ultimate treatment. Indeed, post-operative investigation of such specimens has shown that the tumour infrequently invades the bone despite pre-operative findings of increased scintigraphic image intensity. Enneking assessed the accuracy of bone scans to be in the region of 92% in determining whether or not bone was involved by soft tissue sarcoma. Despite this, he defined bone involvement as the contiguous relationship of bone to the tumour or it's surrounding reactive tissue subsequently verified by pathological examination of the specimen.

False results in this examination occur when the tumour is in the region of areas which may show increased intensity due to other benign causes such as arthritic joints and other non-inflammatory conditions.

Galium-67 citrate scanning can be useful in differentiating between sarcoma and benign non-inflammatory conditions since almost all soft tissue sarcomas, as well as inflammatory masses, will show increased scintigraphic activity, whereas most benign non-inflammatory masses show no increase in tracer activity. Unfortunately, neither galium nor bone scanning is of value in determining the local extent of a soft tissue sarcoma beyond it's involvement with bone.

Detection of Regional or Distant Metastases

Soft tissue sarcomas rarely spread to regional lymph nodes. When present such spread is equivalent to metastatic disease and is always a bad prognostic sign. The only two tumours which do commonly affect regional lymph glands are synovial sarcoma and rhabdomyosarcoma in childhood. Lymphangiography is of limited benefit since, whilst it will occasionally demonstrate metastatic involvement in regional lymph nodes, false positives are common, especially in the lymph glands of the groin.

Clinical examination is probably more helpful than any specific diagnostic imaging technique for the detection of regional lymph node involvement with tumour. Biopsy of regional lymph nodes can be undertaken where doubt exists after clinical examination.

Intravenous pyelograms or barium studies of the colon may be of assistance in the assessment of pelvic or retro-peritoneal tumours which can cause local compression or displacement of viscera with distortion of the normal anatomy seen in these investigations.

The assessment of the extent of any dissemination of the tumour completes the pre-biopsy evaluation of a primary soft tissue sarcoma. Distant spread of this tumour most frequently involves the lung, the liver and bone. Technetium 99m polyphosphate bone scanning illustrate bone metastases. The detection of pulmonary metastases is possible by normal standard chest x-ray (Fig. 3). However, this will only demonstrate relatively large lesions.

Furthermore, the appearance of pulmonary metastases on a standard radiograph often lags behind the development of these lesions in the lung by a considerable period. Standard radiographs are not, therefore, efficient in the early detection of such lesions. Conventional tomography is slightly more sensitive than the standard radiograph but, again, in the early stages of the disease will probably give a false negative result. Computed axial tomography (Fig. 4) is far more sensitive even than conventional tomography [9] and is particularly successful in the detection of peripheral, pleural based lesions. It's high degree of sensitivity does, unfortunately, give a considerable number of false positive results, that is lesions which are subsequently found at operation to be inflammatory in origin rather than malignant.

However, most clinicians prefer an investigation with a higher guarantee of detecting pulmonary metastases at an earlier stage, albeit with a number of false positives, than a less efficient system rendering a significant number of false negative results. The increasing sophistication of computed scanning devices is in-

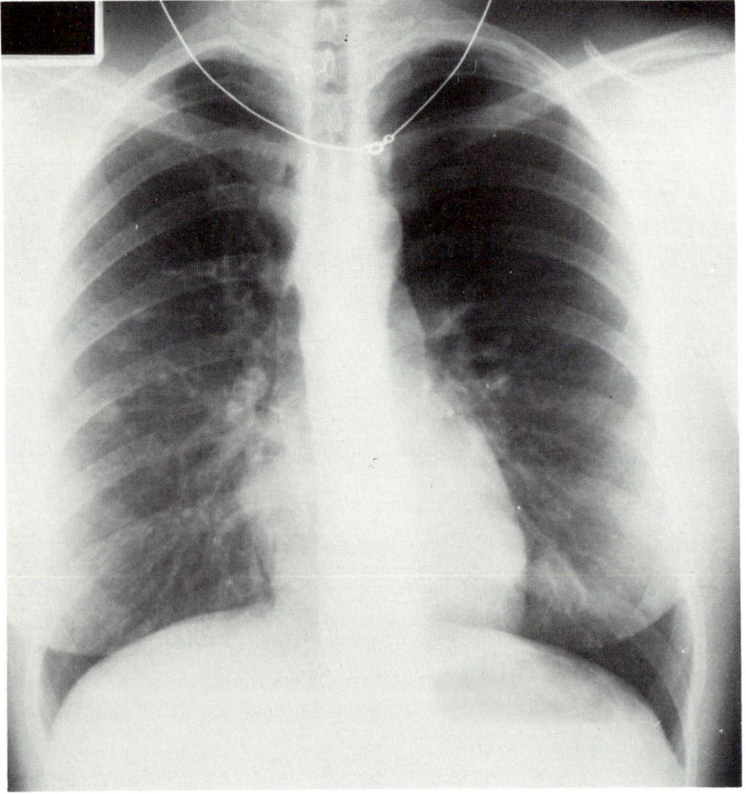

Figure 3. Standard chestfilm showing lung metastases.

creasing the efficiency of the early detection of pulmonary metastases in this disease.

Metastatic deposits within the body of the liver can be detected by ultrasonic scanning of that organ, a test with a high degree of accuracy.

Biopsy

This is the final and most important investigation before definitive treatment. Whilst all other pre-operative investigations are designed to evaluate the local and distant extent of the tumour coupled with it's technical operability; a tissue diagnosis is vital to definitive treatment. Wherever possible the biopsy should be performed by the surgeon who will undertake the definitive surgery. It should never be left to inexperienced junior surgeons nor obtained by another clinician prior to referral. The programmed series of pre-operative investigations are essential in determining the appropriate site for biopsy, the need for open rather than closed

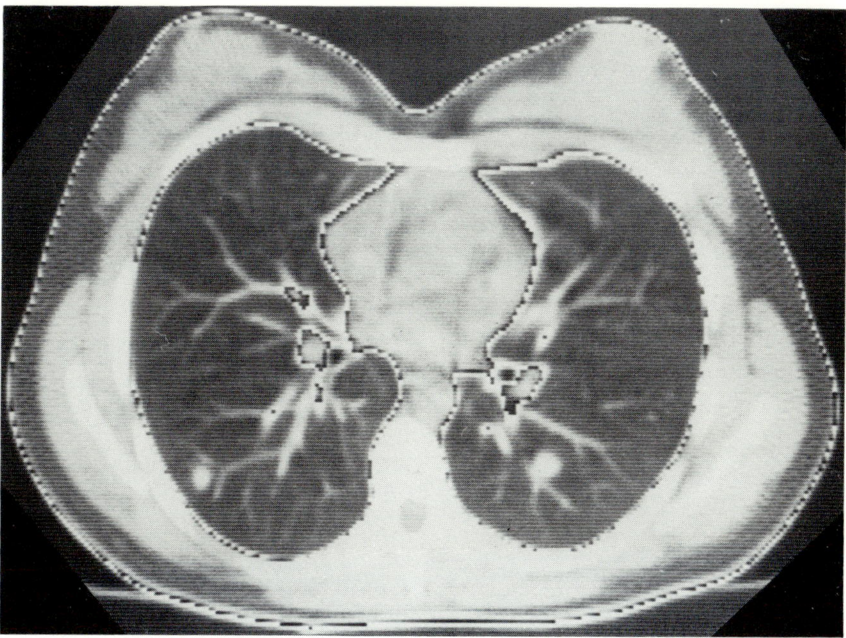

Figure 4. CT-scan of the lungs clearly indicating small metastases in both lungs.

biopsy or, indeed, for excisional rather than incisional biopsy, the advisability of using a tourniquet, the usefullness or otherwise of frozen section diagnosis or special tissue studies coupled with the possibility of immediate operative treatment. Performance of the biopsy should therefore be the final act in the pre-operative investigation of patients suffering from soft tissue sarcomas, since any form of operative interference with the tumour will affect the tissue planes and distort the results of radiographic and scintigraphic studies. Furthermore, the results of those pre-operative investigations may indicate a differential diagnosis before biopsy which will allow a more firm foundation for definitive diagnosis at biopsy.

Most pathologists prefer to make the final definitive diagnosis of soft tissue sarcomas by staining techniques. Frozen section analysis is, in most centres, inaccurate and does not give sufficient information to enable the surgeon to proceed from biopsy to definitive surgery. However, frozen section analysis is useful as an adjunct to stained sections, particularly in identifying the cell of origin through monoclonal antibody studies. In difficult, particularly small, tumours a frozen section analysis will enable the surgeon to ensure that he has obtained a representative biopsy before closure of the wound. Complete pre-operative investigation allows frozen section and standard analysis of the biopsy specimen followed by definitive surgical excision of the tumour if this is feasible or desirable. Whilst this is not widely recommended, since soft tissue sarcomas are a difficult histological group which do not often allow accurate frozen section analysis, biopsy undertaken as the ultimate pre-operative investigation does enable the surgeon to place his biopsy incision at a site which would enable him to continue with definitive surgery in the event of an accurate, confident histological diagnosis on frozen section.

The anatomical site of the biopsy incision is vital to the future surgical management of the patient. It should be based on the differential clinical diagnosis, the extent of the primary tumour as predicted by clinical staging and the site of the tumour in relation to vital structures. After correlating all this information; understanding the principals of limb preservation procedures, standard and non-standard amputation techniques, the surgeon can formulate a surgical plan, placing the biopsy incision in a situation amenable to definitive resection of the tumour with any of those likely potential procedures in mind.

The relative advantage and disadvantage of open and closed biopsy should be clearly understood. Needle biopsy leaves a very small puncture wound which can easily be excised at surgery. It produces only a small amount of bleeding with minimal risk of haematoma formation. There is less likelihood of infection and the procedure is relatively simple. It's greatest disadvantage is that it is always a blind procedure and yields only a small specimen for histological examination. This increases the risk of inadequate tissue sampling and undoubtedly decreases the overall accuracy of the histological diagnosis in a group of tumours which present difficulties in histological diagnosis in any event. Furthermore, whilst it is simple to excise the puncture wound at the time of definitive surgery it is difficult to be sure of excising the needle track along which tumour cells will inevitably have seeded during the biopsy procedure. This can lead to unexpected local recurrence of tumour at the site of surgery. On the other hand, open biopsy requires an incision which must be sufficiently large to enable exposure of the tumour within it's compartment. There is a high risk of haematoma formation, infection and, in particular, dissemination of tumour within the previously normal soft tissues of that and other compartments. A distinct advantage is that a large tissue sample can be obtained and, where indicated, samples can be taken from different areas of the tumour, thus enabling a more accurate histological diagnosis and grading of the specimen. These samples can be selected under direct vision, enabling suspect areas to be closely examined for histological variation within it's overall mass.

Open biopsy remains the procedure of choice in most centres and is certainly preferred by most pathologists carrying out work in this field. The incision should be carefully placed in order that it can be easily excised at the time of definitive surgery. If amputation is contemplated the biopsy incision should fall within the area which is to be sacrificed, allowing sufficient clearance for adequate flaps to be fasioned. In general, longitudinal incisions should be encouraged since transverse incisions are more difficult to excise. Areas of major neurovascular structures should be avoided wherever possible in order to safeguard against their accidental damage or contamination. Seeding of tumour cells in the area of a neurovascular bundle leads to extension of tumour along the neurovascular plane leading to inevitable local recurrence. Care should be exercised in preventing penetration of other, demonstrably normal, muscle compartments since, again, this will attract significant risk of tumour extension. A sharp scalpel should be used throughout the procedure, taking care not to crush the specimen. The incision should be the smallest possible which is compatable with adequate, safe tissue sampling and post-operative haemostasis. In addition to obtaining a specimen of the tumour mass, a biopsy should always be taken from the area of the pseudo-capsule. Wherever possible the tumour should be appraoched through a muscle splitting incision. In the region of the tumour the muscle will become paler in colour. Although there is a considerable variation depending upon the type of tumour and it's vascularity, the sarcoma itself will usually appear grey or white in colour. It usually appears to be well encapsulated. No attempt must be made to dissect the pseudo-capsule either in an attempt to perform a 'shelling out' procedure or to assess it's physical extent. The surgeon must discipline himself to the requisition of a specimen from the tumour. Any attempt at widespread investigative dissection will lead to dissemination of the tumour in that and possibly other muscle compartment. If there has been pre-operative irradiation, tissue which has been irradiated should be avoided as should the central necrotic area of the tumour. These areas provide a poor histological specimen and affects the accuracy of histological diagnosis. Meticulous haemostasis and layer by layer closure of the wound is vital to the patient's future management.

In tumours sited in the peripheral part of a limb, the use of a tourniquet may assist the surgeon in obtaining an accurage biopsy. However, tourniquets should be avoided it at all possible. When used, the limb should never be exsanguinated by compression since this encourages tumour cell embolization. When a tourniquet is used it should always be released prior to closure of the wound in order that meticulous haemostasis can be achieved before closure.

It is essential to recognize that local surgical eradication of this disease depends upon meticulous surgical technique. Definitive surgery should ensure complete local obliteration of macroscopic and microscopic disease. This requires excision of the tumour with a cuff of normal tissue at least 2.5 cm in thickness around the whole of the tumour. The biopsy incision should be regarded as part of that tumour and should be skirted by 2.5 cm of normal skin when performing the definitive surgical incision. If that can not be achieved, ablation of the limb is preferable to the risk of recurrence of tumour at the site of operation. If there is suspicion that microscopic disease remains, particularly after histological examination of the specimen, the site should be irradiated once the wound has healed. Locally recurrent disease should be investigated using the identical programme of investigation except that biopsy is unnecessary. It usually shows a histological grading at least 1 grade more malignant than the initial primary tumour. Excision biopsy by 'shelling out' tumours at the pseudo-capsule interface should be actively discouraged. It inevitably leads to local recurrence of tumour at the operation site.

Conclusion

Surgery is still the only curative method of treating soft tissue sarcomas. It's success depends upon scheduled pre-operative investigation carried out in a logical, organised and disciplined fashion. This will lead to an improvement in the survival rate of patients suffering from this rare but highly malignant disease.

References

1. Enneking W. F., Spanier S. S. and Malawer M. M.: The effect of the anatomic setting on the results of surgical procedures for soft parts sarcoma of the thigh. Cancer 47: 1005 – 1022, 1981.
2. Rosenberg S. A., Suit H. D., Baker L. H. and Rosen G.: Sarcomas of the soft tissue and bone. In: Cancer (de Vita V. T., Hellman S. and Rosenberg S. A., eds) p. 1036, Lippincott, Philadelphia, 1982.
3. Weingrad D. N. and Rosenberg S. A.: Early lymphatic spread of osteogenic and soft-tissue sarcomas. Surgery 84: 231 – 240, 1978.
4. Lindell M. M., Wallace S., de Santos L. A. and Bernardino M. E.: Diagnostic technique for the evaluation of the soft tissue sarcoma. Semin. Oncol. 8: 160 – 171, 1981.
5. Bernardino M. E., Jing B., Thomas J. L., Lindell M. M., Zornoza J.: The extremity soft-tissue lesion: a comparative study of ultrasound, computed tomography and xeroradiography. Radiology 139: 53 – 59, 1981.
6. De Santos L. A., Goldstein H. M., Murray J. A. and Wallace S.: Computed tomography in the evaluation of musculoskeletal neoplasm. Radiology 128: 89 – 94, 1978.
7. Berger P. E. and Kuhn J. P.: Computed tomography of tumors of the musculoskeletal system in children. Radiology 127: 171 – 175, 1978.
8. Hudson T. M., Haas G. H., Enneking W. F. and Hawkins I. F.: Angiography in the management of musculoskeletal tumors. Surg. Gynecol. Obstet. 141: 11 – 21, 1975.
9. Pass H. I., Dwyer A., Makuch R. and Roth J. A.: Detection of pulmonary metastases in patients with osteogenic and soft-tissue sarcomas: The superiority of CT-scans compared with conventional linear tomograms using dynamic analysis. J. Clin. Oncol. 3: 1261 – 1265, 1985.

3. Staging of soft tissue sarcomas

David E. Markham

The heterogeneity of soft tissue sarcomas has for a long time hampered the development of a clinical staging system despite the well recognized importance of such a system. Staging provides the possibility of an optimal treatment planning, of comparing treatment methods with regard to their results, and of quality control of information for analysis. The soft tissue sarcomas can be grouped together to allow sufficient numbers to develop a staging system, because histology has been found to be less important than histological grade.

In 1968 the Task Force of the American Joint Committee for Cancer Staging and End Results Reporting devised a staging system for soft tissue sarcomas based on the TNM system of the UICC but also including histological grade (Table 1) [1]. They distinguished low, moderate and high grade soft tissue sarcomas, based upon criteria such as cellularity, cellular pleomorphism and mitotic activity. In recent years grading has been defined more optimal (see chapter 1). Regardless of cellular differentiation etcetera, some tumors are considered highly malignant. The AJC system also takes notice of the fact that involvement of bone and/or neuromuscular structures has a poorer prognosis than regional lymph node metastases, and that tumour size should not, in itself, dictate the method of surgical treatment.

Russel et al. [2] used the AJC system to review 1215 cases of thirteen types of soft tissue sarcomas and found that stage was well related to survival indicating the usefulness of the system.

Enneking [3] has formulated a different surgical staging system for use in both bone and soft tissue sarcomas (Table 2). Because it is less cumbersome than the AJC system it has gained popularity amongst surgeons. However, histological grade is only subdivided into high and low grade, reducing the accuracy of this important factor. Stage I are low grade sarcomas subdivided into A and B by anatomical location. A indicating tumor restricted to one anatomical compartment and B indicating extra-compartmental tumor spreading, i.e. in more than one anatomical compartment or where the intercompartmental barrier is invaded. Stage II are high grade sarcomas and can also be subdivided into A and B, whilst

Pinedo, H. M., Verweij, J (eds) Clinical Management of Soft Tissue Sarcomas
© *1986 Martinus Nijhoff Publishers, Boston. ISBN 0-89838-808-2. Printed in The Netherlands.*

Table 1. Schema for staging soft tissue sarcomas by T, N, M and G.

T	Primary tumor
	T_1 Tumor less than 5 cm
	T_2 Tumor 5 cm or greater
	T_3 Tumor that grossly invades bone, major vessel, or major nerve
N	Regional lymph nodes
	N_0 No histologically verified metastases to regional lymph nodes
	N_1 Histologically verified regional lymph node metastasis
M	Distant metastasis
	M_0 No distant metastasis
	M_1 Distant metastasis
G	Histological grade of malignancy
	G_1 Low
	G_2 Moderate
	G_3 High

Stage I		
Ia	$G_1T_1N_0M_0$	Grade I tumor less than 5 cm in diameter with no regional lymph nodes or distant metastases
Ib	$G_1T_2N_0M_0$	Grade I tumor 5 cm or greater in diameter with no regional lymph nodes or distant metastases
Stage II		
IIa	$G_2T_1N_0M_0$	Grade 2 tumor less than 5 cm in diameter with no regional lymph nodes or distant metastases
IIb	$G_2T_2N_0M_0$	Grade 2 tumor 5 cm or greater in diameter with no regional lymph nodes or distant metastases
Stage III		
IIIa	$G_3T_1N_0M_0$	Grade 3 tumor less than 5 cm in diameter with no regional lymph nodes or distant metastases
IIIc	Any $GT_{1-2}N_1M_0$	Tumor of any grade or size (no invasion) with regional lymph nodes but no distant metastases
Stage IV		
IVa	Any $GT_3N_{0-1}M_0$	Tumor of any grade that grossly invades bone, major vessel, or major nerve with or without regional lymph node metastases but without distant metastases
IVb	Any $GTNM_1$	Tumor with distant metastases

stage III includes distant metastatic tumor of any grade. This means that this staging system does not take account of lymph node involvement. Although this system enables the surgeon to select the correct definitive surgical procedure, the neglectance of lymph node involvement and the less detailed grading result in a less accurate use for analysis of end result studies.

Table 2. Enneking's surgical staging system.

Stage I-A	Low grade intracompartmental lesion without metastases
Stage I-B	Low grade extracompartmental lesion without metastases
Stage II-A	High grade intracompartmental lesion without metastases
Stage II-B	High grade extracompartmental lesion without metastases
Stage III	Any grade with metastases

A third staging system for soft tissue sarcomas (Table 3) has been developed by Hajdu [4]. However he only differentiates low and high grade tumors and the system does not recognize anatomical compartments. Whilst it is appreciated that superficialy located tumors have a more favourable prognosis than those which are situated in deeper tissues, this is only one factor in the overall consideration of the grade of malignancy. Tumor size and site are not always reliable criteria upon which to base ultimate surgical procedures in this disease. For these reasons the system of Hajdu is only of limited usefulness and can not be applied to analysis of the results of treatment.

Conclusion

An accurate staging system for soft tissue sarcomas is essential to our understanding of the disease and the effectiveness of its treatment. Only by the use of such a system can the effects of treatment be monitored and modified, leading to a

Table 3. Hajdu's staging system.

	Good prognostic signs	Bad prognostic signs
Size	Small – less than 5 cm	Big – more than 5 cm
Site	Superficial – not beyond superficial fascia	Deep – beyond superficial fascia
Histologic grade	Low – hypocellular – much stroma – minimal necrosis – good maturation – mitosis $<5/10$ HPF	High – hypercellular – minimal stroma – much necrosis – poor maturation – mitosis $>5/10$ HPF

more effective success rate in eradication of this disease.

Soft tissue sarcomas are rare and, as a group, represent a complex series of tumours. An understanding of their behaviour would be enhanced by the universal use of one staging system in order that all tumours worldwide could be compared in relation to their behaviour and their response to treatment. Whilst the system of Russell is the more complex of three staging systems in general use, it's complexity is not such as to significantly deter surgical oncologists from it's utilization. It has distinct advantages over the other two systems in terms of histological grading. It's universal use should be encouraged in both surgical and pathological circles.

References

1. Russell W. O., Cohen J., Enzinger F., Hajdu S. I., Heise H., Martin R. G., Meissner W., Miller W. T., Schmitz R. L. and Suit H. D.: A clinical and pathological staging system for soft tissue sarcomas. Cancer 40: 1562 – 1570, 1977.
2. Russell W. O., Cohen J. Edmonson J. H., Enzinger F., Hajdu S. I., Heise H., Martin R. G., Miller W. T., Schmitz R. L. and Suit H. D.: Staging system for soft tissue sarcoma. Semin. Oncol. 8: 156 – 159, 1981.
3. Enneking W. F., Spanier S. S. and Goodman M. A.: Current concept review. The surgical staging of musculoskeletal sarcoma. J. Bone Joint Surg. 62-A: 1027 – 1030, 1980.
4. Hajdu S. I.: Pathology of soft tissue tumors. Lea and Febiger, Philadelphia, 1979.

4. Surgical treatment of soft tissue sarcomas

Myron Arlen, M. D. and Ralph C. Marcove, M. D.

Introduction

The management of soft tissue sarcomas of the lower extremity can be considered to represent the standard by which we plan for the management of most of the sarcomas arising elsewhere in the body. These tumors not only are found to occur more frequently in the lower extremity, which adds to the importance of this site, but in terms of management the techniques employed here can be, and frequently are translated to other body sites. The use of muscle group dissection needed to surgically encompass most of the lesions that are encountered, and the techniques for vessel dissection especially in the region of the groin, can be paralled for the arm-axillary region and may even be extended to the muscles and blood vessels of the head and neck. We feel that the ability to become familiar with the natural history of, and master the surgery needed to control soft tissue sarcomas arising in the lower extremity, offers a broad base from which to understand and manage most of the sarcomas found at other sites.

Soft tissue sarcomas of the lower extremity

It is generally accepted that most malignant tumors arising in and around muscle groups, tend to have local infiltration and as such, set the stage by which we approach them surgically. Soft tissue sarcomas tend to infiltrate through a pseudocapsule and insinuate into adjacent fascial planes, making margins of resection difficult to define by gross examination or by frozen section. The findings of giant cells in the periphery of the tumor and in surrounding tissue usually represents coalesced muscle nuclei destroyed by tumor invasion. Adequate resection usually requires that the fascia be resected along with the tumor mass.

At secondary resection, further removal of surrounding tissue and regional nodes when indicated has often revealed the presence of residual microscopic disease. If failure to remove the tumors completely has taken place then such inade-

Pinedo, H. M., Verweij, J (eds) Clinical Management of Soft Tissue Sarcomas
© *1986 Martinus Nijhoff Publishers, Boston. ISBN 0-89838-808-2. Printed in The Netherlands.*

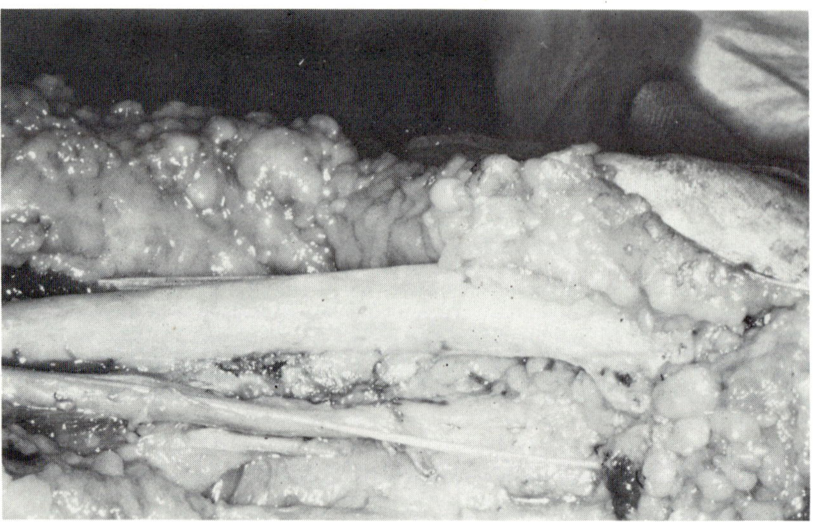

Figure 1. Exposed femur after extended quadricepts resection for liposarcoma.

quate resection will usually be followed by tumor spreading centripetally along the fascial planes of the extremity, but not necessarily within a given muscle group. If the primary occurred in the upper thigh then it is probable that retroperitoneal structures will in due time be reached and invaded as a result of invasion through psoas region or obturator membrane. Other sarcomatous lesions may extend deeply around muscle bundles eventually reaching down to the periosteum of bone (Figs. 1, 2). Some sarcomas, as they spread within the extremity, can occasionally involve lymphatic channels and invade regional lymph nodes; most others must be considered in terms of their potential vascular and neural invasion spreading to distant sites along these pathways.

While the importance of proper histologic classification remains of primary concern, of equal importance is proper assessment of deeply placed lesions which frequently can be misinterpreted or overlooked.

Clinical identification is usually defined only after the lesion has reached quite extensive proportions (Fig. 3). Any assymetry in an extremity which has recently appeared should therefore be considered as potentially malignant and does require investigation. The presence of a lesion existing for several years does not exclude malignancy.

If soft tissue sarcomas are deeply located in the leg, their margins are frequently adjacent to the periosteum of femur, tibia or sacrum; here the major mass of the tumor will be found to lie under such structures as the gluteus, quadraceps or soleus.

In rare instances, we have also noted such lesions occurring in the region of interosseous membrane between radius and ulna or tibia and fibula. It is improba-

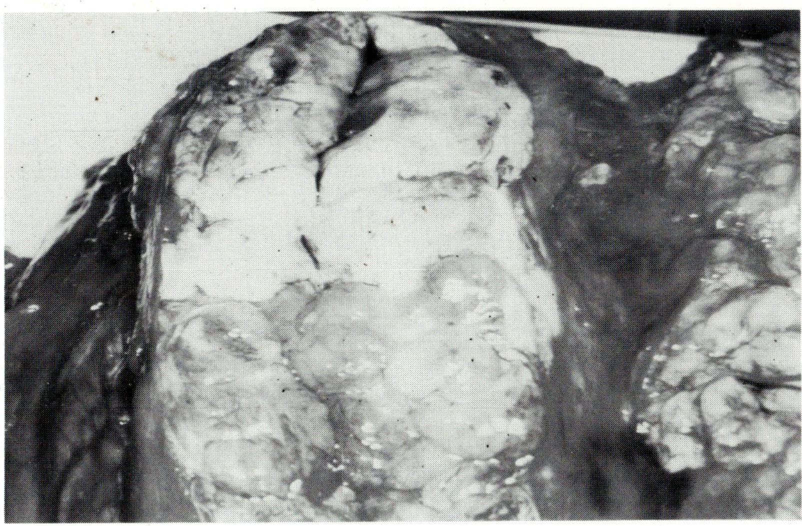

Figure 2. Specimen of liposarcoma with central groove where lesion had wrapped around femur.

ble that such tumors could have been easily identified early in their clinical course, since most were asymptomatic during their initial growth phases. By careful questioning, one can come to realize that symptoms in many of those patients were actually present for more than one year prior to diagnosis.

Sudden swelling of a limb may be a clue to vascular infiltration and blockage, especially seen with epithelioid sarcoma.

One of the major factors in making a decision as to the type of surgery to be employed for any soft tissue sarcoma, as mentioned, has to be based on the diagnosis obtained by biopsy (see chapter 2). If the tumor is found to be malignant, the new incision line for resection must ellipse the previous incision site which may have been seeded by tumor cells. It is important to plan the direction of the incision so that it will not only encompass the biopsy site, but include those underlying structures which must be removed. The direction of the incision should also be aimed along the most common pathway for metastasis, so that the optimum degree of resection can be performed to include fascial planes that may have been involved.

Angiography is important in the workup of patients with extremity sarcomas that have been proven by biopsy (see chapter 2). It may reveal a pattern of extension not appreciated on clinical examination as well as the possibility of blood vessel involvement (encasement), or displacement. Major vascular feeders can be defined which may have to be ligated prior to definitive resection. Vascular displacement and infiltration by tumor can be noted, suggesting that possible vascular grafting may be needed.

In those instances where superficial infiltration of adventitia of the adjacent

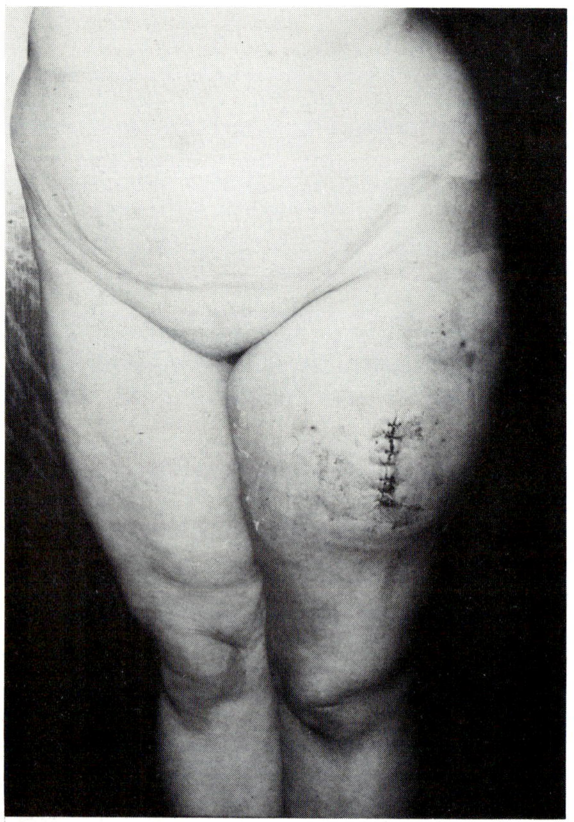

Figure 3. Expansive rhabdomyosarcoma filling entire left thigh.

vessels may have occurred by low grade tumors, the tumor can still be resected with careful dissection of the blood vessels using sharp scalpel removal.

In the surgical approach for any of the deeply seated sarcomas, the amount of skin and extent of muscle and subcutaneous tissue to be resected is important. After creating an elliptical incision around the site of biopsy, to assure that the biopsy tract is included in the resection, relatively thick skin flaps should be raised as long as the tumor does not appear to infiltrate the subcutaneous tissues. Under these circumstances, 2−4 cm of normal skin can be removed with the biopsy site and underlying subcetaneous tissue. One must constantly palpate the lesion without visualizing it as the deeper structures are transected. One may find the tumor mass extending into planes not appreciated by superficial palpation. The extent of the deeper structures to be included can then be modified so that additional surrounding normal tissue can be included around the tumor. Normal muscles should surround the lesion. When the tumor mass is greater than 5 cm in diameter, the muscle group or groups should be traced to an divided at their origins

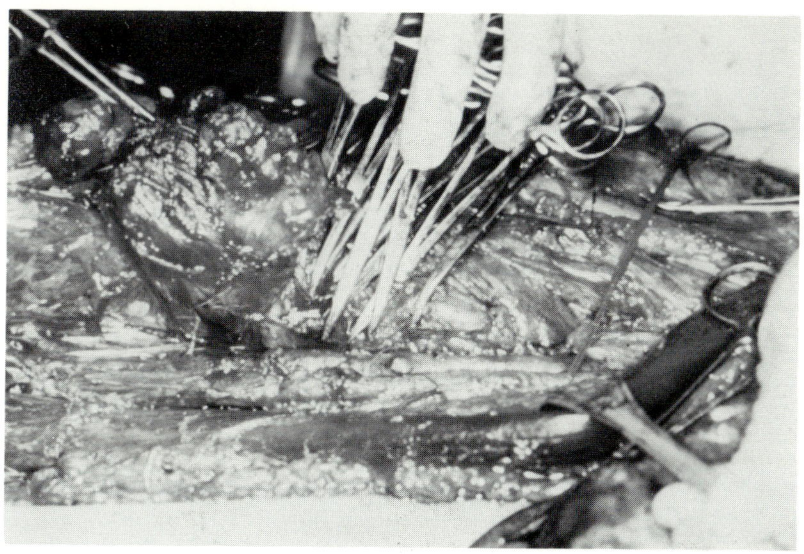

Figure 4. Resection of a highly vascular lesion off femoral vessels.

and insertions. At this time if bone is near the pseudo-capsule of the tumor it too can be resected. A complete set of (Marcove modified Guepar) knee or hip resection prosthesis makes bone or joint substitution easier and can be utilized on the spot as resection needs require.

Complete control of blood supply is essential during such surgery with perforating tumor vessels being isolated at their origin and controlled with hemoclips or silk ligatures (Figs. 4, 5). When dissecting a lesion of the mid thigh, it might be necessary to identify the femoral artery by extending the incision superiorly to the groin.

Once defined, the artery can be dissected toward the tumor mass to insure that the lesion can be freed properly from the primary blood supply to the leg in a situation where blind dissection could have resulted in vascular injury. As the perforating vessels which enter the tumor are identified, hemoclips can be used to secure them at their origin and these structures can then be transected. In most instances, if the angiogram and CAT scan suggest that the vessel is free of tumor then adequate dissection to retract major vessels from the tumor site can usually be accomplished. If evidence is found of vessel invasion by tumor, then an adequate dissection cannot be accomplished and resection of the main arterial supply may be needed with insection of a vascular graft. In many instances when there is extensive disease about the neurovascular pedicle then amputation must be considered.

The result of surgical resection for lower extremity sarcomas has been reported in several large series. In each, the lower extremity has appeared to be the most prevalent site for the occurrence of tumor. Shiu [11], in a review of 297 cases seen

50

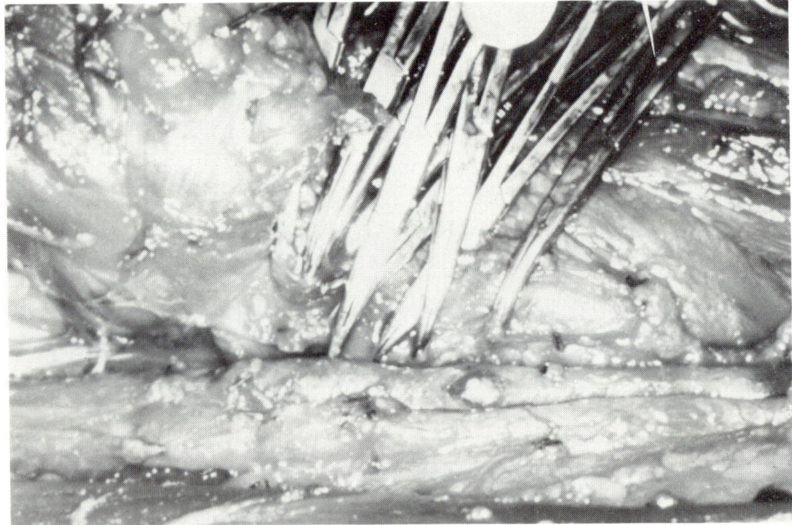

Figure 5. Resection of a highly vascular lesion off femoral vessels.

at Memorial Hospital between 1949 and 1968, described what appears to be the well founded experience of most surgeons. 'Local inadequate resection has resulted in the highest rate of local recurrence'. In terms of the distribution of tumors within the lower extremity, the thigh was the most common location with 211 cases being seen. The leg itself was the second most frequent site with 60 cases arising there. The foot contained 16 of the neoplastic tumor masses. One might anticipate such a distribution in terms of the extent of soft tissue present at each site that is potentially at risk. Even though tissue volume was greatest in thigh and normal muscle mass surrounded the tumor to the greatest degree, poor survival rates occurred in the thigh. This was possibly due to the closer proximity to pelvis and a somewhat greater delay in diagnosis.

The bulky normal tissue surrounding the tumor in the thigh may also have led to a longer delay in clinical recognition, especially when the tumor arose in the deeper muscle planes. In terms of tumor size, the largest lesions to be treated occurred in thigh, both in anterior and posterior muscle compartments. We have noted similar findings not only with regard to delay in diagnosis, but also in terms of hesitation in making the decision to treat, since many tumors produced expansion within the thigh very subtly and a diagnosis of a malignant neoplasm was not initially made. In some patients, on the contrary, the lesions were extremely bulky and we were faced with the decision to do surgery in borderline situations. These patients had been turned down with only hemipelvectomy being offered to them as the treatment of choice. Many of these large bulky tumors did not initially appear to metastasize, but had seeded vascular and fascial planes early. Such tumors tend to grow, reaching enormous proportions prior to the onset of therapy. Even at this time, wide muscle group dissection has been possible for many of these patients.

As we have learned, the presence of a large tumor size does not always mean that amputation will be necessary. Rather, the findings of extension of tumor to inguinal ligament, vessel invasion and bone involvement are more of an indication for the possible need for amputation. With more sophisticated approaches many of these barriers are now being taken down and extremities are being saved.

Liposarcoma

In contrast to the frequently seen lipomas of the extremity which are the primary tumor masses to be encountered and are easily discernable from surrounding structures, the infiltrating lipomas are uncommon and are found within the musculature of the upper as well as the lower extremities.

They are difficult to totally excise, because of extension within muscular planes and are therefore prone to recurrence. Rarely, infiltration becomes so extensive that muscle dysfunction may result or sensory changes appear due to pressure on nerve trunks. The vascular component of these tumors is inconspicuous and consists mostly of capillaries. Lesions to be excluded from the diagnosis of infiltrating lipoma, include intermuscular lipoma, benign lipoblastomatosis, hibernoma, intramuscular lipoma and spindle cell lipoma. Hibernomas occur more commonly in the subcutaneous tissue of the back. The infiltrating angiolipomas appear firm, fixed and are frequently associated with pain and swelling. Histologically, a prominent vascular pattern can be found and may be reflected by severe bleeding at the time of surgical resection.

If the tumor that has been resected represents a liposarcoma, then the incidence of recurrence and even possible metastasis can be fairly high. As a small fatty tumor enlarges in size, especially if one has been watching it for a long period of time, the possibility that malignancy is present increases. A rule that one should bear in mind, is that when dealing with any fatty tumor larger than 5 cm in diameter, where enlargement appears to be continuing, one must biopsy it in order to prove the actual histologic makeup. For many fatty tumors, areas of malignant transformation are not usually uniform, so that random biopsy may not show the true nature of the lesion (Fig. 6). Only after adequate sampling has been accomplished or if the lesion has been removed completely, can one rely on histologic verification of malignancy or benignity.

At Memorial Hospital, approximately 20% of the lower extremity soft tissue sarcomas are represented by liposarcomas. They have a particular predilection for the inner thigh and the region of the popliteal space.

The liposarcomas are usually painless masses beginning in the deep soft tissues and frequently attain significant size without ulcerating the skin. Grossly, the tumors may resemble fatty tissue especially in the lipoblastic tumors. When cut

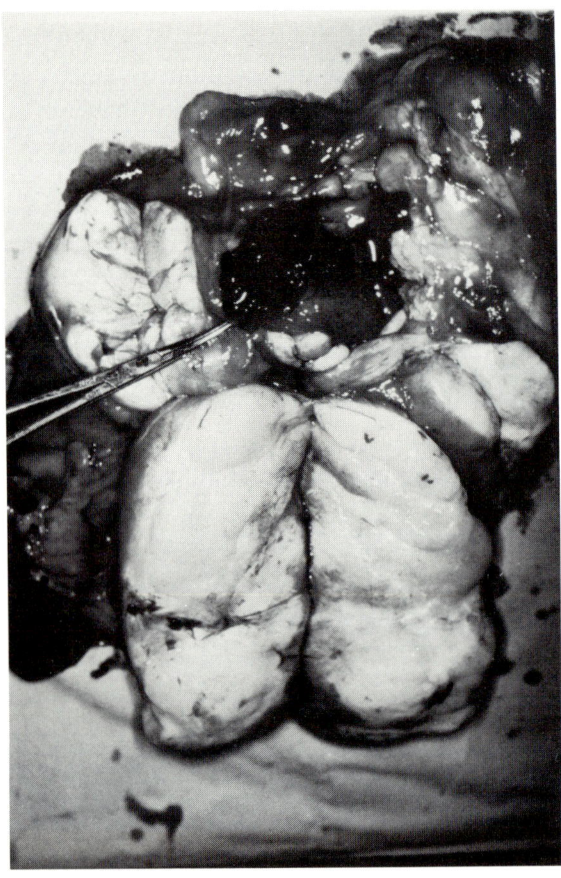

Figure 6. Surgical specimen showing different areas of malignant growth in one tumor.

into, if yellow oily fluid runs out, the diagnosis of liposarcoma should be made. Angiographically, these tumors show vascular patterns inversely related to the degree of differentiation. Low-grade, well differentiated tumors are usually vascular, compared to the more pleomorphic lesions. Enzinger and Winslow [5], in 1962, had given figures of a 53 to 85% survival rate depending on the histologic type for the liposarcoma. The histologic patterns of the recurrence are usually similar to the primary tumor for most reported series. In a few instances, higher grades of neoplastic recurrence may be seen. At Memorial Hospital, about 25% of the recurrent tumors had been reported to develop less differentiated forms with each recurrence. In spite of the presence of a bulky tumor and extensive infiltration seen with many lesions, major structural infiltrations such as skin, blood vessels, nerves and bone are not common initially for the primary tumors. When involvement does occur it should be handled accordingly, i.e. liposarcomas in close proximity to bone should not be treated by subperiosteal resection, but rather by bone resection with adjacent tumor included. Many of the thigh tumors tend to be expansile and not infiltrative. This leads to an initial displacement rather than invasion of surrounding structures which is one of the reasons why en-bloc muscle groups dissections can be curative. The liposarcomas of the extremity follow a distribution pattern of recurrence with the lower extremity being most frequent site, followed by upper extremity and then retroperitoneum.

Recurrences that appear following failure to widely resect tumor may be noted to reappear at intervals over a protracted period ranging from 5 to 20 years without showing signs of distant metastasis.

Lymph node metastases are rare, but do occur with liposarcoma. Malignant lipomatous tumors tend to spread to lung frequently presenting with peppering of the pleural surface of the lung and diaphragm, rather than as discreet cannonball lesions.

In those instances where tumor does approximate bone, and where good margins of resection are possible, one may choose to do an en-bloc resection, including femur with prosthetic replacement. This procedure has been described by Marcove [8], for osteosarcomas and has been extended to many soft tissue sarcomas where the potential for cure is feasible should the femur be included as part of the operation.

Discrete, innocous appearing nodular subcutaneous masses may in reality be malignant tumors, so that sound clinical judgement is necessary should one decide to delay their biopsy.

Malignant fibrous histiocytoma

Malignant fibrous histiocytoma represents one of the more common tumors to be found in the lower extremity. The primary clinical finding seen with this type of tumor, as for most tumors occurring in the thigh, is the presence of a discrete mass. Approximately 10% of the patients described have noted poorly localized pain. Thirty percent have also been found to have osseous changes on x-ray, including lytic areas of the cortex as well as periosteal region. Kearney [6], reported results seen in 167 cases of this type of tumor treated at the Mayo Clinic between 1947 and 1976. Eighty five occurred in the lower leg and 60 were found in the thigh; 8 were seen about the knee, 15 in the leg and 2 on the feet. The tumors were classified as superficial or deep; the former were found entirely in the subcutaneous tissue and deep lesions arose in or involved underlying muscle groups.

In the thigh, 41 of 60 tumors were deeply placed. The reverse was noted for most of the sites below the knee. The fibrous tumors were most commonly seen with the giant cell variant; myxoid and inflammatory components were found to a lesser degree. Wide resection was the obvious treatment of choice. Of the 36 patients that had been referred with a history of complete excision and where en-bloc resection was then performed, 15 showed residual tumor microscopically.

Among patients with superficial tumors, the local recurrence rate after complete excision was 71%; for deeper tumors it was 41%. One would suspect that complete excision of the superficial group was inadequate compared with the surgery that was employed for deeper placed tumors. In both groups we would have to assume that the en-bloc operation probably could have more comprehensively removed the tumor should proper neurovascular dissection have been performed. Patients with lesions situated above the knee appear to do worse in the long run than those that are distally placed. Tumors proximally situated in the thigh were found to be more frequently associated with metastasis to sites such as lungs, regional nodes and retroperitoneum. Ekfors et al. [4] reported 38 cases of malignant fibrous-histiocytoma of the extremity among 246 sarcomas. Again the thigh was the most frequent site for these tumors to occur in. The predominant modality of treatment was excision followed by radiation therapy. In 17 patients there were one or more reoccurrences and in 21, evidence of metastatic spread. Eleven patients survived more than 5 years. The number of recurrences suggested that the primary operation was usually not adequate.

Synoviosarcoma

For those patients who have had a proven diagnosis of synoviosarcoma, most of the lesions have appeared in the region of the thigh or about the knee (60 – 70%). In the young patient who presents with a history of trauma to the extremity and a mass showing diffuse calcification, one should consider the possibility that the lesion is a synovioma. The trauma of course is unrelated to causative factors but seems to call the patients attention to the existence of the lesion. Biopsy, again is essential to rule out the presence of a benign traumatic mass. Once the diagnosis of synovioma has been established, wide resection with removal of surrounding muscle groups is employed as we do with luposarcoma and malignant fibrous-histiocytoma. Approximately 5 – 10% of these lesions may spread to regional nodes and for this group of patients en-continuity regional node dissection should be employed, especially when a large lesion approximates groin or the suggestion of nodal involvement is present. The incidence of lymph node metastasis may be lower than what has been reported if one eliminates neglected cases of epitheloid sarcomas which have been confused with malignant synovioma.

Leiomyosarcoma

Smooth muscle tumors such as leiomyosarcoma do appear on occasion in the extremities and when seen usually are of venous origin. We have advocated that tumor masses in the region of the groin be removed by an en-bloc approach including the nodes in the saphenofemoral junction; this would obviate any problem that might necessitate further re-exploration of this region, even if the tumor proved to be a lymphoma. For many of the tumors arising in this region, removal of the superficial nodes above the saphenofemoral junction may only reveal hyperplastic changes.

In actuality, the true pathology may reside deeper in the unresected nodes. Should an extensive mass of nodal tissue be present, removal of the complete cluster of nodes sitting on the femoral vein, might define the actual nature of the pathologic process.

Malignant schwannoma

Among the lesions to be considered in the lower extremity, those arising from nerve structures also have been an important role in the clinical spectrum of neoplastic disease. Storm et al. [15] evaluated 20 patients with malignant schwannoma. Fourteen of these patients had associated neurofibromatosis. Analysis of the clinical data collected suggests that there is an excellent correlation between tumor size, cellular pleomorphism and mitotic activity in terms of survival for this tumor. In this series, 4 lesions occurred in the proximal and 5 in the distal leg. For this group of tumors, local excision alone resulted in a two-thirds local failure rate.

The ability to define neurogenic malignancies in general and the malignant schwannoma in particular may be difficult. Morphologically, the tumors must be defined on a clinical ground as arising in nerve sheath. The incidence of association of Von Recklinghausen's disease is generally under 50%, but may in some series, reach two-thirds of the cases. The findings of pain and enlargement due to a possible nerve mass, especially when associated with Von Recklinghausen's disease, should alert one to the chance of possible malignant transformation in a pre-existing benign nerve tumor. Most of the malignant schwannomas arise from major nerve trunks, such as brachial plexus, sciatic nerve and sacral plexus. They may be confused histologically with fibrosarcoma, monophasic synovioma, leiomyosarcoma and as such, close association with nerve trunks or plexuses should be clearly defined when considering neurogenic sarcoma.

Rhabdomyosarcoma

Rhabdomyosarcomas can produce large masses in the thigh and lower leg (Fig. 7). Such tumors may be found to have such extensive involvement on angiography and CAT scan that there appears to be no possibility of performing a muscle group dissection. In some instances other treatment modalities can reduce the lesion to one that is surgically managable without the need for amputation. Occasionally, a small nodular mass can be present in the thigh, which on biopsy proves

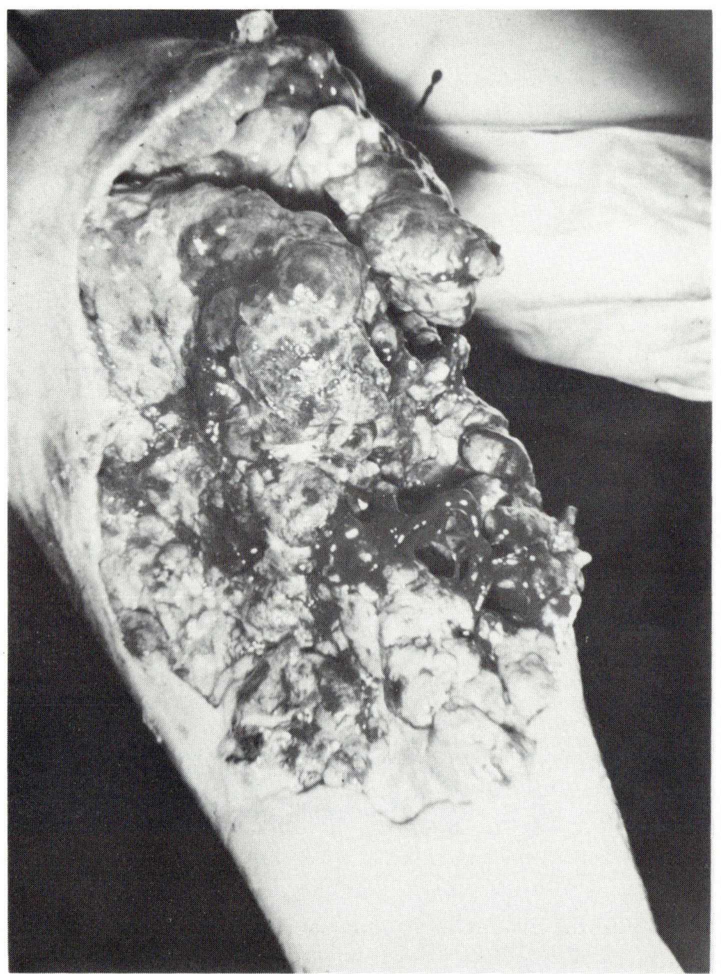

Figure 7. Extensive pretibial rhabdomyosarcoma.

to be rhabdomyosarcoma (Fig. 8). Here, wide resection can be accomplished without too much difficulty. Fig. 8 shows a small superficial multinodular mass that had been initially excised and proved on pathological examination to be rhabdomyosarcoma. The lesion went untreated for several months. The patient was referred for definitive treatment, which consisted of wide resection down to the sartorius. In order to be sure that this tumor was completely removed, the femoral vessels were identified adjuvant to the sartorius and dissected free of surrounding overlying muscles. Fig. 9 shows the tumor sitting on the surface of the muscle with good margins of resection having been achieved.

In many instances, the first clinical presentation of rhabdomyosarcoma of the lower extremity is the appearance of an ill-defined swelling. This can also be seen

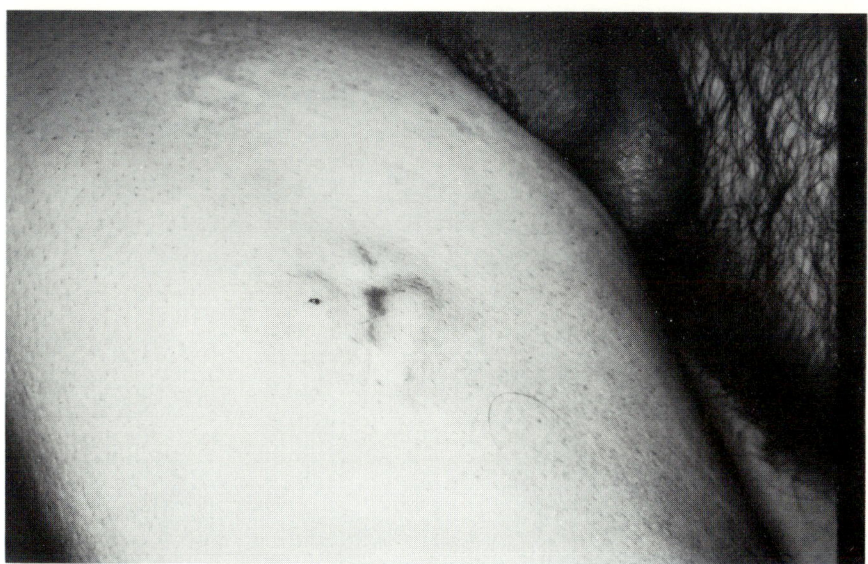

Figure 8. Small recurrent rhabdomyosarcoma of the mid right thigh.

in cases of liposarcoma where deep muscle groups are involved. If there is any question as to the possibility of resectability when lesions are exceedingly large, then preoperative therapy sometimes may allowe preservation of the extremity.

Fibrosarcoma

Fibrous tissue tumors are also among the more common lesions seen. Among the 64 patients with fibrosarcoma followed between 1937 and 1969, Bizer [1] noted 11 cases distributed in the upper extremity and 15 in the lower extremity with 15 occurring on the trunk. Seven of the patients (11%) demonstrated microscopic regional metastasis. Fifty patients underwent initial surgical resection, 20 having been treated by local resection. In 74% of these patients local recurrence developed. Twenty were initially treated by radical resection with a 30% incidence of local recurrence. In several patients, radical tumor resection necessitated amputation because of the size and position of the fibrosarcoma. The absolute 5 year survival rate for all cases was 44%.

Soft tissue sarcomas of the trunk

The presence of sarcomas arising on and about the superficial structures of the trunk, chest and abdominal wall are well defined. These lesions are not as frequently encountered as those we find appearing on the extremities. It is essential

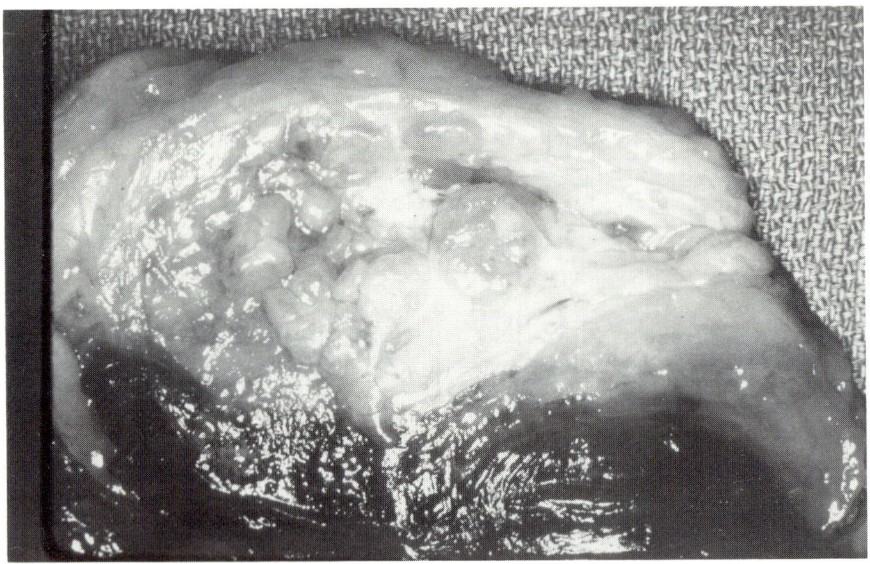

Figure 9. Specimen showing tumor sitting on resected sartorius muscle.

that when they do appear, they be identified correctly and be treated in an equivalent fashion, since failure to do so may result in an uncontrollable situation even if a tumor is known to be low-grade and with a high potential for cure.

Similar to extremity lesions, truncal lesions require that they be widely resected with adequate margins of normal surrounding tissue if there is going to be any potential for possible cure. Such a resection may require incision into the underlying deep fascia and muscle of the chest wall and may even include a portion of the rib cage. If underlying chest wall needs to be resected, than stability can be achieved with marlex mesh.

The mesh should be folded over at its edges, (doubled), and sutured first with interrupted marlex or prolene sutures placed into bone or periosteum. A second layer of running sutures is used for approximation of the edges of the prosthesis to surrounding fascia which in effect produces a taut-firm layer of mesh. In the chest wall in order to prevent paradoxial motion, methyl methacrylate can be applied between layers of marlex to achieve rigidity of the mesh. For abdominal wall lesions, adequate surgical management may necessitate resection of a considerable portion of abdominal musculature, underlying parietal peritoneum and periosteum of pelvic bones when necessary. In certain instances, large tumors may actually penetrate through peritoneum, necessitating visceral contents to be included with the resection.

In the Memorial Hospital series of abdominal wall sarcomas, six patients required resection of underlying viscera. This especially holds true where a large lesion has penetrated through fascia. At this time the aggresiveness of the lesion can be anticipated and one must be ready not only to resect abdominal wall with probably reconstruction but one should anticipate that intestinal viscera will be involved. Among the 22 lesions that were found to be abdominal wall sarcomas 12 were eligible for evaluation. Four had been untreated and eight previously treated. Two of the four survived 5 years; 4 of the eight previously treated recurrent tumors reappeared again after an additional surgical attempt. The defect that remains is usually reconstructed by inserting marlex mesh by which stability is easily achieved and hernias are obviated. Marlex mesh is most often used for replacement of musculo-fascial defects, though other synthetic meshes, of fascia and tensor fascia lata have also been tried. Under most circumstances skin flaps can be mobilized to cover the prosthetic mesh. At times this is not possible and a proper myocutaneous flap should be employed guaranteeing thickness and vascularity to the pedicle.

The deltopectoral flap is one of the few that can be raised without underlying muscle adhering to the flap since it is supplied by direct cutaneous vessels fed from the internal mammary chain. Other flaps such as the pectoralis myocutaneous and latissimus flap are fed by large vessels i.e. thoracoacromial and thoracodorsal vessels. The thoracroacromial artery enters the pectoralis flap leaving the second portion or the axillary artery and entering the muscle 2 cm medial to the coracoid process and 2 cm inferior to the clavicle. A pedicle based at the clavicle and extending just medial to the nipple can be raised with a sizable paddle of skin. When an aggressive approach is taken early, even high-grade malignancies may be managed satisfactorily this way.

Fibrous tumors

For fibrous tissue tumors, the size and clinical appearance of a tumor does not always characterize the behavior of the neoplasm in question. It is apparent that there is a wide spectrum of tumors of fibrous tissue origin beginning with the well known keloid and progressing on to plantar and palmar fibromatosis and then to the desmoid tumor and dermatofibrosarcoma protuberans, a tumor commonly involving chest wall. Eventually, fibrosarcomas are seen at the other end of the spectrum of such tumors. The clinical pattern set by any of these lesions does not appear to be wholly related to any existing microscopic pattern; rather the behavior of such tumors tends to be associated with the relative position it occupies within the spectrum of fibrous tissue responses. Knowledge, therefore, of the relationship that exists within this spectrum is important in predicting the clinical behavior and deciding treatment that is needed.

In the past, the significance of cellular activity among the fibrous tissue tumors have often been misinterpreted with early invasiveness or metastasis predicted yet never occurring. Similarly, a histologically benign appearing lesion may have already invaded locally or even metastasized.

Local recurrence is frequently a common finding in dermatofibrosarcoma. More commonly, among the large nodular masses that we find on the anterior abdominal and chest wall, desmoids are of prime consideration. These growths denote the presence of a tendinous tumor. Brasfield and DasGupta [2] described a series of 38 cases seen at Memorial Hospital. A high preponderance of females to males, 3 to 1, was found. Two patients were under 10 years of age, the mean age for the group was 30. Eighteen patients in this series had tumors occurring in the rectus abdominis and the external oblique muscle of the abdominal wall; two occurred in the internal oblique and transverse and two in transverse abdominis. The majority presented with a painless anterior abdominal wall mass. Only 4 patients complained of any abdominal symptoms. Pregnancy could be directly linked to 6 cases, usually appearing after the second pregnancy and with the tumor mass arising in the anterior rectus sheath. This site may represent the effect of stretching of muscle fibers or the effect of trauma. Cases of abdominal desmoids have been seen after repeated traumatic episodes to the anterior wall. Surgical scars were definitely associated with the initiation of tumor in 6 of the patients. The differential diagnosis of the abdominal wall masses should include: 1) fibrosarcoma, the most important tumor to be considered; 2) neurilemomma, which lesion is usually softer and seen more commonly with von Recklinghausen's disease; 3) dermatofibrosarcoma, which usually presents as a more nodular lesion and 4) lipoma, a tumor most frequently found to be subfascial in origin.

The findings of an abdominal wall mass in a patient recently pregnant usually signifies the presence of an abdominal desmoid tumor. There is little question that these tumors are under the influence of hormones and that the pregnant state offers the optimum milieu for this tumor to grow. Since the desmoid tumor is considered by many to represent a low-grade fibrosarcoma, wide resection with adequate, (at least 4–5 cm), margins of resection are needed to prevent the typical patterns of local recurrence that are seen. The treatment in general is well defined and follows the tenet for management of essentially all sarcomas.

The problem of dealing with recurrence in this tumor is quite common, because all too often the lesion has not been considered malignant and adequate resection is not performed. This tumor on reappearance requires further resection than initially performed, even if a major portion of the abdominal wall or chest wall is to be removed. Replacement by means of mesh and use of rotation pedicle flap for skin coverage is always needed. Adequate resection is usually curative. Only 4 of 35 patients in the Memorial series developed recurrence. Distant metastases is unusual and may only rarely been seen. The more common patterns for recurrence are usually seen in those lesions which appear higher in the spectrum of fibrous tissue tumors, such as dermatofibrosarcoma protuberans.

Malignant fibrous histiocytoma

Malignant fibrous histiocytoma, a common sarcomatous lesion of the extremity may also be found arising as a primary tumor mass on the chest and abdominal wall. Occasionally it has been reported to arise within breast tissue. Among the 53 cases described by Obrien and Stout [9] the breast was the site of origin in 5.

Langham et al. [7] reported a similar lesion appearing in the left breast. Seven previous cases aside from Stouts were described. Three occurred in women with a history of other tumors or previous radiation. One developed in association with cystosarcoma phylloides and 3 arose following radiation for carcinoma of the breast. Some form of modified mastectomy appears in order when these tumors are found to arise in breast. In the case reported by Tsuneyoshi and Emjoji [13] the patient had 4 recurrences over a period of 4 years with eventual freedom of disease at 68 months. Metastases are unusual and axillary node dissection probably is not indicated unless nodes are palpable. Malignant fibrous histiocytic lesions arising in the skin have also been reported to involve breast. More localized resection can be offered for these cases in contrast to the therapy required with the deep MFH of breast.

References

1. Bizer L. S. Fibrosarcoma; Report of 64 cases. Am. J. Surg. 121: 586 – 587, 1971.
2. Brasfield R. D., DasGupta T. K. Desmoid Tumors of the Anterior Abdominal Wall. Surgery 65: 241 – 246, 1969.
3. Eilber F. R., Morton D. L., Eckart J., Grant T., Weisenburger T. Limb Salvage for Skeletal and Soft Tissue Sarcomas. Cancer 53: 2579 – 2584, 1984.
4. Ekfors T. O., Rantakokko V. An Analysis of 38 Malignant Fibrous Histiocytomas in the Extremities. Acta Path. Microbiol. Scand. Sect. A 86: 25 – 35, 1978.
5. Enzinger F. M., Winslow D. L. Liposarcoma; A Study of 103 Cases. Virchows Arch. Path. Anat. 335: 367 – 388, 1962.
6. Kearney M. M., Soule E. H., Ivins J. C. Myxoma of Somatic Soft Tissues. Mayo Clin. Proc. 48: 401, 1973.
7. Langham M. R., Mills A. S., DeMay R. M., O'Dowd G. R., Grathwohl M. S., Horsley J. S. Malignant Fibrous Histiocytoma of the Breast. Cancer 54: 558 – 563, 1984.
8. Marcove R. C., Abou-Zahr K. En-Bloc Surgery for Osteogenic Sarcoma. Bull. N.Y. Acad. Med. 60: 748 – 758, 1984.
9. O'Brien J. E., Stout A. P. Malignant Fibrous Xanthoma. Cancer 17: 1445 – 1455, 1964.
10. Prior S. T., Sisson B. S. Dermal and Fascial Fibromas. Ann. Surg. 139: 453 – 000, 1954.
11. Shiu M. N., Castro E. G., Hajdu S. I., Fortner J. G. Surgical Treatment of 297 Soft Tissue Sarcomas of the Lower Extremity. Ann. Surg. 182: 597 – 602, 1975.
12. Storm F. K., Eilber F. R., Mirra J., Morton D. L. Neurofibrosarcoma. Cancer 45: 126 – 129, 1980.
13. Tsuneyoshi M., Emjoji M. Postirradiation Sarcoma (Malignant Fibrous Histiocytoma) Following Breast Carcinoma. Cancer 45: 1419 – 1423, 1979.

5. The Role of Radiation Therapy in the Treatment of Soft Tissue Tumors

George A. Trivette, Jane Grayson and Eli J. Glatstein

Introduction

The last two decades have witnessed a significant change in the role of radiation therapy in the treatment of soft tissue sarcomas. Although surgery remains the primary treatment for most soft tissue tumors, there has been a marked increase in the use of combined modality therapy for localized tumors, employing less radical surgery in combination with radiation therapy. The goals of this combined approach include improved local control as well as reduced anatomic and functional deficit. The role of chemotherapy in the treatment of high grade sarcomas will be discussed in other chapters.

Although a number of early papers documented objective responses of soft tissue tumors to radiation therapy [1, 2, 3], radiation was considered for many decades to be merely a palliative modality in these tumors [4, 5]. Certainly in the era prior to megavoltage equipment, skin toxicity limited the ability to administer the relatively high doses of radiation necessary for the primary treatment of soft tissue tumors. As early as 1951, Cade [6] reported on the successful use of wide local excision and radiation therapy in sarcomas. Significant advances in the combined modality approach were made at M. D. Anderson Hospital (MDAH) in the 1960's [7, 8]. Since that time, many institutions have reported on the successful integration of radiation and surgery in soft tissue tumors [9, 10, 11]. Recent data from the prospectively randomized National Cancer Institute (NCI) trial [12] comparing amputation to limited resection plus postoperative irradiation in high grade sarcomas of extremities support the comparable local control rate with these two approaches. The rationale for combining the two modalities is that radiation can control microscopic extension of tumor into adjacent normal appearing tissue following surgical removal of the obvious gross tumor with a generous margin. The extent of the resection is still controversial, ranging from wide local excision to muscle group resection. Radiation can obviously encompass major nerves, vessels, and bones, which would be approachable surgically only with amputation in many instances. Functional results with this approach have generally been

Pinedo, H. M., Verweij, J (eds) Clinical Management of Soft Tissue Sarcomas
© *1986 Martinus Nijhoff Publishers, Boston. ISBN 0-89838-808-2. Printed in The Netherlands.*

good. Collaboration from the initiation of treatment with a concerned physical therapy department is extremely important.

In addition to the use of postoperative irradiation in soft tissue tumors, many patients have been treated with preoperative irradiation [13, 14], intersitial irradiation [14, 15], intraoperative radiation therapy, [16], and radiation therapy combined with intra-arterial chemotherapy [17]. These techniques are presently being investigated with ongoing studies to see if any of these approaches offer advantages over postoperative irradiation.

There are also a number of reports of irradiation alone [18] or in conjunction with radiosensitizers [19] in patients in whom a surgical option was not available. Although data from the Massachusetts General Hospital (MGH) demonstrate that results for local control with radiation therapy alone are not comparable to the excellent data from combined modality treatment, local control and cure can be achieved in perhaps 30% or greater of patients so treated. The recent NCI findings of surprisingly good local control in patients with unresectable sarcomas treated with irradiation and halogenated pyrimidines are intriguing and suggest that further investigation is warranted. Additional investigation is also being carried out to establish the role of neutron beam irradiation in the primary treatment of sarcomas.

This chapter reviews the current status of the use of radiation therapy in the treatment of soft tissue tumors. Emphasis is placed on extremity sarcomas which constitute greater than 50% of the soft tissue tumors. The approach for truncal and head and neck tumors employing surgery and radiation therapy follows basically the same principles. Anatomic considerations in these sites often make the technical problems more difficult both for the surgeon and the radiation oncologist. Attempts are made, as with extremity tumors, to ultilize a series of conedown fields to minimize surrounding normal tissue toxicity.

The role of radiation therapy in low grade and benign soft tissue tumors is discussed. The same combined modality approach used in local therapy of high grade tumors is very effective in preventing local relapse in low grade tumors. Major questions remain as to the extent of the surgical procedure which is necessary and in which circumstances radiation therapy is required.

It is apparent that as methods are increasingly effective in achieving local control in soft tissue tumors, expanded efforts will be needed to find improved treatment of microscopic- and gross metastatic disease in these patients and to further improve survival rates.

High grade extremity lesions

Soft tissue sarcomas invade aggressively into surrounding tissues and have a high frequency of early hematogenous dissemination especially to the lung. The local aggressiveness of soft tissue sarcomas results in the development of a *compression zone* surrounded by a *reactive zone* of fibrous and connective tissue [20]. These form a pseudocapsule which is unlike a true capsule since it only gives the appearance of circumscription. Fingers of tumor can extend to and through the pseudocapsule along nerve fibers, muscle bundles, fascial planes, and blood vessels. Therefore, local recurrences have been reported up to 12 cm from apparent gross tumor. However, tumors localized within a muscle compartment rarely invade through the fascia into adjacent soft tissue except in advanced cases. However, violation of these planes by surgery can facilitate local extension.

The rationale for the use of radiation therapy as an adjuvant to conservative surgery can be developed by looking at the frequency of local failure with different surgical techniques for high grade sarcoma. Definitions of the different techniques by Enneking and his associates[1] are based on the surgical margin:

1) *Incisional biopsy* involves removal of a small portion of tissue usually for diagnostic purposes which could lead to local contamination.
2) *Excisional biopsy* of the tumor and pseudocapsule without margin which potentially leaves fingers of tumor at the margin.
3) *Wide excision* of the tumor and pseudocapsule with a variable margin depending upon the philosophy of surgeon. This leaves potential microscopic aggregates of tumor which were not encompassed in the procedure.
4) *Radical resection* of the lesion and normal tissues in continuity with it by at least one uninvolved anatomic structure. The muscular structures, nerves, vessels, and bone in the compartment are removed. Therefore, an amputation is often required to do this procedure.

Thus, using Enneking's definitions, the expected local recurrence would be 100% with incisional biopsy, 80–100% with excisional biopsy, around 50% with wide excisional biopsy, and 10–20% using radical local resection. Examples of local recurrence rates in different series are shown in Tables 1 and 2. Eighty percent of the local recurrences will occur by 2 years [22].

The purpose of adding radiation therapy to surgery is to allow for conservation of the anatomic site without amputation. Numerous reports have shown that soft tissue sarcomas are responsive to irradiation [8, 26, 30, 31]. It is felt that a dose of approximately 6000 cGy combined with wide local excision should be enough to control microscopic disease. The radiation can be given either preoperatively or post operatively depending upon the preference of the surgeon and radiation oncologist. Suit and his associates at Massachusetts General Hospital prefer preoperative irradiation since they can restrict their treatment volume, increase resectability, and decrease the chance of autotransplantation from exfoliation [8]. At the NCI, we prefer postoperative irradiation which allows for exact pathologic classification, direct physical assessment of tumor extent, and sterilization of exfoliated cells without the increased morbidity of operating in an irradiated bed. Table 3 shows that conservative surgery plus irradiation results in local control equivalent to radical resection (i.e., amputation).

Table 1. Local recurrence following local or wide local excision. (Adapted from Leibel et al. (21).)

Author (Ref.)	Type of surgery			
	Local excision		Wide local excision	
	# of patients	# of patients with local recurrence (%)	# of patients	# of patients with local recurrence (%)
Cantin et al. (22)	n.d.	n.d. (42)	n.d.	n.d. (30)
Gerner et al. (23)	58	54 (93)	25	15 (66)
Markhede et al. (24)	19	14 (74)	n.d.	n.d. ($-$)
Martin et al. (25)	218	168 (77)	n.d.	n.d. ($-$)

n.d. (no data).

Table 2. Local recurrence following radical local excision or amputation. (Adapted from Leibel et al. (21).)

Author (Ref.)	Type of surgery			
	Radical local excision		Amputation	
	# of patients	# of patients with local recurrence (%)	# of patients	# of patients with local recurrence (%)
Leibel et al. (26)	11	3 (27)	16	2 (13)
Rosenberg et al. (27)	n.d.	n.d.	83	0 (0)
Shiu and Hajdu (28)	194	57 (29)	185	14 (8)
Simon and Enneking (29)	25	3 (12)	29	6 (21)

n.d. (no data).

Table 3. Local recurrence with conservative surgery and radiation therapy. (Adapted from Leibel et al. (21).)

Author (ref.)	# of patients	Dose (rad)	# of patients with local recurrence (%)
Leibel et al. (26)	29	5,000 – 7,500	3 (10)
Lindberg et al. (8)	300	6,000 – 7,500	67 (22)
Rosenberg et al. (27)	128	6,000 – 7,000	12 (9)
Suit et al. (30)	110	6,000 – 6,800	13 (12)
Suit et al. (30)*	60	6,400 – 6,600	8 (14)

* Pre-op XRT.

There are several specific contraindications to limb sparing surgical resection which include:

1) A lesion so extensive that the margins of resection will be grossly positive.
2) Gross invasion of a joint.
3) Extensive involvement of multiple compartments of the extremity.
4) Invasion of crucial vessels beyond the scope of a vascular graft or reconstruction.

In the experience of the NCI, only around 10% or less of the patients will have these contraindications.

If none of the above contraindications are present, then a combined approach can be attempted. The goal of the surgery at the NCI is wide excision of tumor which is compatible with good function and does not compromise the ability to give adequate radiation therapy. Others prefer only an excisional biopsy [30, 32]. However, we feel that the chance of local control is optimized if only microscopic residual disease needs to be irradiated.

When planning radiation therapy there are eleven basic steps which should be followed to obtain a good functional result. They are:

1) Attend the surgery if possible or discuss with the operating surgeon the precise site of origin, areas of extension, residual tumor, etc.
2) Immobilize the extremity or cast it in order to assure reproducibility of daily set-ups in order to increase the chance of local control, as well as decrease morbidity (See Fig. 1).
3) Avoid turning the patient over since rotation around a major joint can occur in more than one plane. If the total length of the field is greater than can be achieved with a single field, treat isocentrically with pairs of matching fields with the match line moved 1 cm every 1000 cGy. Another method of smoothing out the dose at the match line is the use of a gap wedge [33]. The divergence and sharp penumbra of linear accelerator beams can cause significant morbidity due to random set-up errors. The gap wedge reduces the nonuniformity in the matching region by creating a wide pseudo-penumbra.
4) Define the tumor volume using the surgeon's description, preoperative physical exam, computerized tomograms, etc. One should encompass the full anatomic compartment and usually the muscle completely. Individualized blocks should be made in order to optimize the treatment volume.
5) If necessary, angle the portals in order to encompass all the clips placed at surgery.
6) Wire out the complete extent of the scar. If possible, the portal should strike the scar tangentially to boost the scar. Wedges or tissue compensators may be used to optimize dose distribution. If this is not possible, then tissue equivalent bolus should be used over the scar to increase the dose (See Fig. 2a).
7) In order to assure optimal function and minimize lymphedema, spare a strip of the extremity from direct radiation. Severe fibrosis with decreased func-

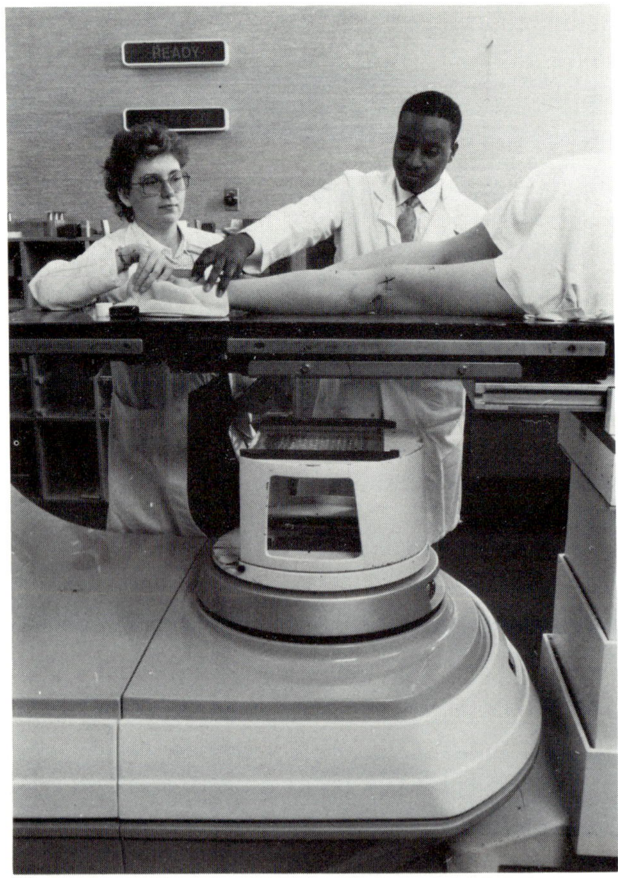

Figure 1. Patient with a synovial cell sarcoma of the right polpiteal fossa who is placed in a foot cast each day to allow for exact daily reproducibility for precision treatment.

tion, pain, and edema can occur with circumferential irradition.

8) Attempt to exclude major joints from radiation if the surgery permits. However, if the scar crosses the joint, exclude a portion of the joint to prevent a frozen joint later on (See Fig. 3).

9) Have the patient begin physical therapy before surgery if possible, throughout treatment, and after treatment in order to maximize the functional result. The value of active physical therapy cannot be overestimated.

10) Use a dose of 6000 cGy or more to the tumor volume at 180 to 200 cGy per day, five days per week. At the NCI, we use 4500 cGy for potential microscopic disease at 180 cGy per fraction, 5 days per week to a large field. An additional 1800 cGy in 10 fractions is then delivered to the area at highest risk for residual tumor for a total dose of 6300 cGy (See Fig. 3).

11) Use shrinking field technique to minimize the volume receiving the highest dose to decrease morbidity (See Fig. 3).

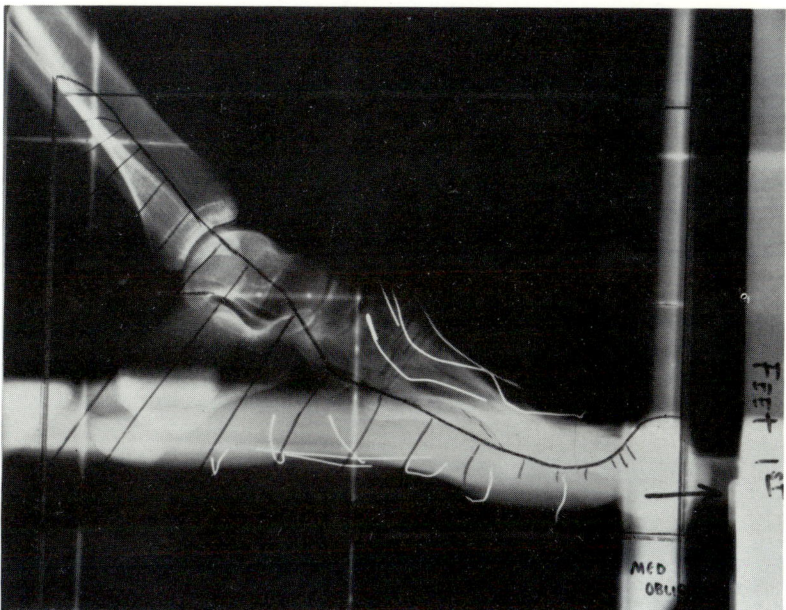

a

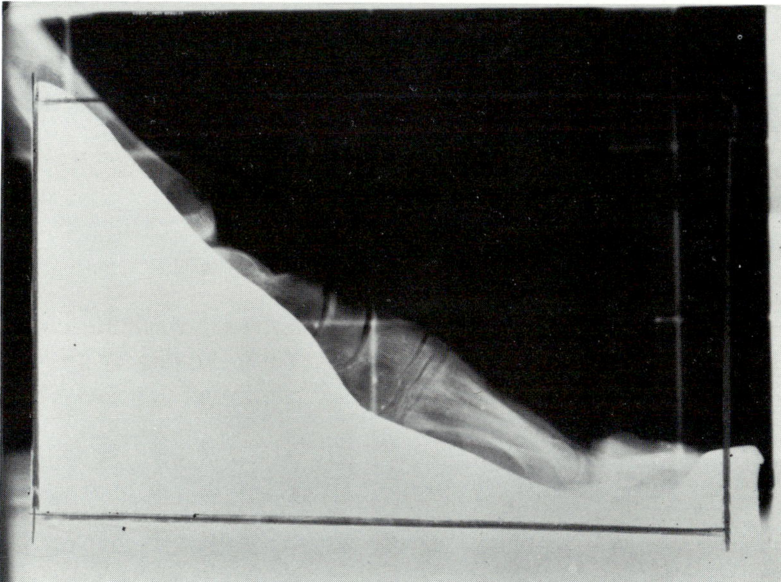

b

Figure 2. a. Simulation film of a patient with a fibrosarcoma of the extensor surface of the foot. Lead wires were used to mark the initial tumor and sole of the food. In addition, circular lead markers were placed at the nails to block them from treatment. The field was rotated to allow adequate coverage of the treatment volume as well as to tangent the scar to bolus it. b. Portal film prior to treatment to show how individual blocks are used to maximize treatment and decrease morbidity by preventing circumferential irradiation of the foot.

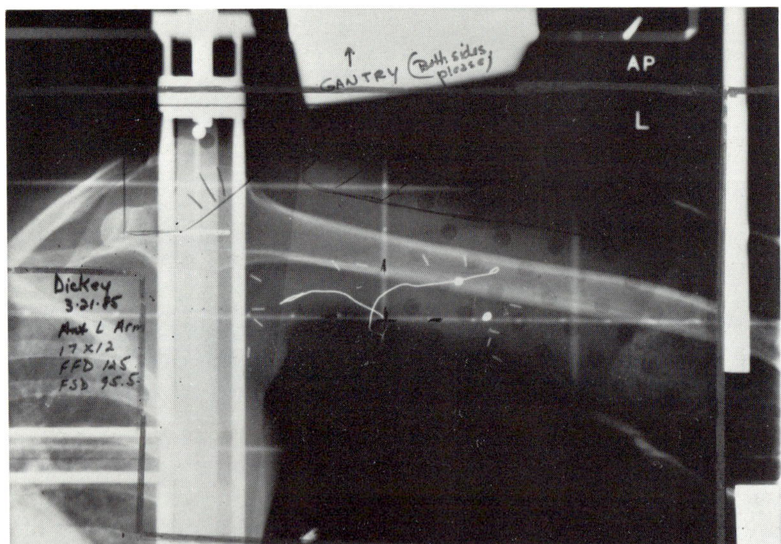

Figure 3. Patient with a Synovial cell sarcoma of the left upper arm. a. Simulation film encompassing the clips with a generous margin which was treated to 4500 cGy. Please note that a portion of the joint was blocked out of the field. b. Simulation film of a conedown field after 4500 cGy for 1800 cGy to encompass the area at highest risk. The decreased field length and an enlarged block protect the shoulder joint from treatment to prevent the morbidity of a frozen joint.

These steps should enhance the chance of local control as well as permit a good functional result. For more detailed descriptions of NCI treatment techniques for different extremity sites, see reference 34.

High-grade retroperitoneal lesions

Retroperitoneal soft tissue sarcomas are rare tumors constituting only 10 to 15% of the soft tissue sarcomas [35]. Therefore, only a few large cancer centers accrue enough of these patients to report their treatment results. Both local control and survival are lower for retroperitoneal soft tissue sarcomas than for extremity soft tissue sarcoma. There are several reasons for this. First, retroperitoneal sarcomas tend to reach enormous size before they are clinically apparent. Secondly, extensive local retroperitoneal resections are difficult due to morbidity; typically the margins of resection are positive for tumor and the surgery is less than a complete resection. Finally, biopsying an extremity lesion is easily done without contamination. However, biopsying a retroperitoneal sarcoma can lead to peritoneal and retroperitoneal contamination [36], a problem which we believe to be underestimated.

In 1981 Cody et al. [19] reviewed 158 patients treated at Memorial Hospital from 1951 to 1977. In patients who underwent complete resection without adjuvant therapy, the local recurrence rate was 77%. This rate is consistent with local failure associated with local excision in extremity soft tissue sarcomas. The use of adjuvant radiation after complete resection increased the five year survival (30% vs 53%) and disease free survival (17% vs 33%). However, it was not statistically significant. There were few five year survivors in patients with partial excision with or without adjuvant chemotherapy and radiation therapy.

In 1984 Tepper et al. [38] reviewed 23 patients, 17 treated with curative intent and 6 treated palliatively, from Massachusetts General Hospital which had been treated between 1971 and 1982. The 17 patients treated curatively were given 4900 to 6900 cGy postoperatively or primarily. Local control was 71% (5/7 patients) with complete resection, 57% (4/7 patients), with incomplete resection, and 33% (1/3 patients) with no resection. The actuarial 5 year survival was 54%. Higher doses of radiation increased local control with 33% (2/6 patients) local control with less than 5000 cGy, 0% (0/5 patients) local control with 5000 to 6000 cGy, and 83% local (5/6 patients) control with greater than 6000 cGy. They concluded that local control and survival were highest with complete resection and high dose radiation therapy. Presently, they are looking at preoperative and intraoperative irradiation to increase their resectability and local control since complete resection and postoperative irradiation still have a high local failure rate.

At the NCI, we have been conducting a randomized trial between surgery and postoperative irradiation for 5400 cGy vs surgery with intraoperative irradiation therapy (IORT) for 2000 cGy (See Fig. 4) and postoperative irradiation for an ad-

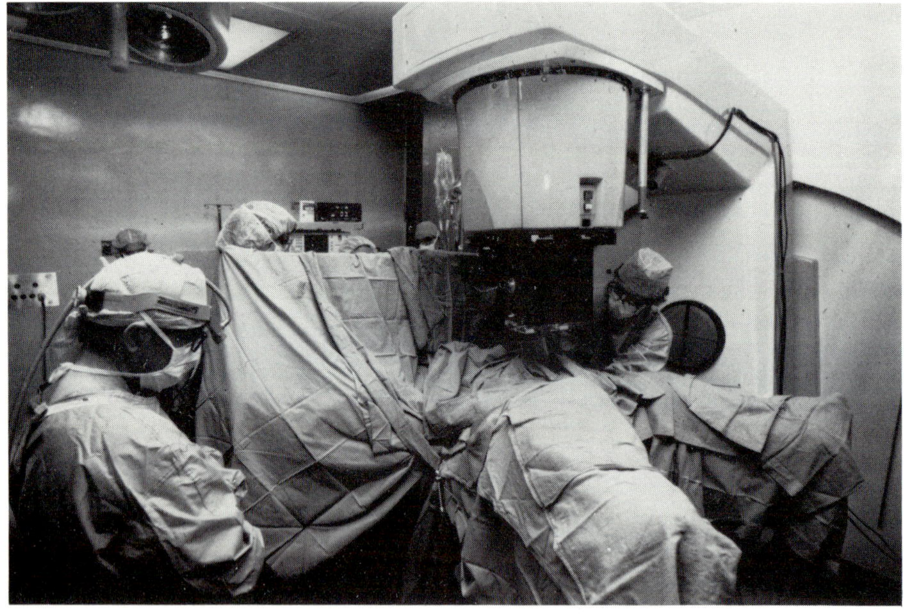

Figure 4. Shows patient during intraoperative procedure with the electron cone being positioned carefully by the physician to allow for exact coverage of tumor bed with the treatment.

ditional 4 500 cGy. Twenty patients were treated with surgery (19 gross resection and 1 no resection), IORT, and postoperative irradiation [16]. Tumors were all greater than 10 cm and intraoperative radiation fields covered 50% or more of the retroperitoneum. Two patients died postoperatively, one with sepsis and another with pulmonary embolus. Of the 18 patients surviving surgery, IORT, and postoperative radiation, the actuarial 3 year survival was 73% with median survival of 44 months. Twelve of the 18 patients (67%) have remained disease free for 6 to 41 months. Local control has been achieved in 14 of 18 patients (78%). Complications included three patients with peripheral neuropathies related to radiation, one vascular insufficiency of the lower extremity from thromboembolism, one late radiation enteritis requiring surgical correction, one pancreatic pseudocyst, and one patient with a superficial skin burn. In our control arm with surgery and postoperative radiation for 5 400 cGy (data unpublished), the local control and survival are not significantly different. There were fewer complications. The most common pattern of relapse on both arms has been intraperitoneal seeding, outside the retroperitoneum. The study is continuing since the number of patients are small and the follow-up is too short to make a final judgment concerning possible benefit of IORT.

Benign and low grade soft tissue tumors

The soft tissues of the body can give rise to benign as well as to malignant tumors. As with high grade sarcomas, an extensive classification based on presumed cell of origin exists for benign and low grade soft tissue tumors [39, 40]. Although identification of the tissue of origin is often less difficult in these well differentiated tumors, considerable controversy over pathologic classification may occur. In addition, establishing a pathologic grade for many of these tumors is also problematic.

The definition of low grade sarcomas and benign soft tissue tumors is quite controversial (chapter 1; [41 – 42]).

Knowledge of histologic grade has important implications in selecting appropriate therapy in soft tissue tumors. Histologic grade is generally accepted as the most important prognostic variable in soft tissue sarcomas [8, 41, 42, 44]. This appears to be true for local recurrence and metastatic spread as well as survival [24, 26, 41, 45]. While treatment of high grade sarcomas must address both local and systemic disease, benign and low grade sarcomas present mainly a problem of local control. The distinction between aggressive benign soft tissue tumors and low grade sarcomas is probably also an important one, although this is not accepted universally.

Although benign tumors may recur locally many times and even result in death from failure to achieve local control, they are considered non-metastasizing growths with rare exceptions. In contrast, true sarcomas, even of low grade, do metastasize with a finite frequency and local recurrence may significantly decrease ultimate survival [24, 22, 46, 29]. Because of the small number of low grade tumors in any given series of soft tissue sarcomas, this is difficult to evaluate accurately.

In considering the benign soft tissue tumors, the majority are successfully treated by simple excision [47]. Others, however, exhibit extremely aggressive local behavior and have a higher likelihood of local recurrence after excision. In these lesions, wide local excision with removal of adequate surrounding tissue is more critical. It is in this group of tumors that the role of radiation therapy should be considered. Because the cells of these low grade tumors divide and express cell death very slowly, it should be emphasized that one must wait much longer to see regression than for most other neoplasms.

The most common of these aggressive soft tissue tumors are in the category of benign tumors of fibrous origin. They are classified with the fibromatoses and include those designated as desmoid tumors. Desmoids arise from fascial sheaths and musculoaponeurotic structures and can occur in any anatomic location. Their ability to infiltrate deeply into surrounding structures has been well documented [48, 49, 50, 51]. The anatomic site of the tumor appears to influence the ability of surgery alone to prevent local recurrence, with abdominal tumors most accessible to surgical removal. Abdominal desmoids tend to occur more frequently in females, particularly of child-bearing age, although the relationship of abdominal desmoid tumors to pregnancy in unclear. Several early series report a significant frequency of local recurrence in abdominal desmoids [48, 52]; more recent reports treated with wide local excision, including underlying fascia, report excellent local control. In the series from Memorial Sloan Kettering Cancer Center [50], recurrence is reported in only 1 of 29 patients who could be treated with 'adequate' surgery for primary abdominal desmoids. Data from the University of Helsinki confirms this with 2 of 34 recurrences in completely removed abdominal desmoids [53].

However, unlike the successful results in abdominal desmoids, the local recurrence in extra-abdominal or inadequately excised tumors ranges from 20 to greater than 60% [48, 49, 54, 55, 56]. The role for radiation therapy in such extra-abdominal desmoids is unclear. Aggressive surgical therapy in a series from Memorial Sloan Kettering Cancer Center [49] on extra-abdominal desmoids, 42 of whom were seen for initial treatment and 30 with locally recurrent tumor, resulted in a 25% (18/72) rate of lcoal recurrence. In this series, of patients eligible for five year follow-up, 4/5 patients with amputation were controlled, 2/2 with muscle group resection, and 27/45 (60%) with wide excision achieved local control. Radiation therapy has not generally been used in desmoid tumors; one recent report [53] suggests no benefit to radiation, although only 6/80 patients received any radiation. Several early surgical series included small numbers of patients with inoperable disease controlled with radiation therapy [48, 51]. Three recent reports [57, 58, 59] review a number of patients with incomplete excision, unresectable tumors, or an unacceptable surgical option who received radiation therapy for desmoid tumors. Of patients with gross tumor masses, control was achieved in 8/10 (MGH), 7/8 Joint Center for Radiation Therapy (JCRT), and 9/13 University of California, San Francisco (UCSF, tumors of greater than 10 cm), for total control of 24/31 (77%) in this unfavorable subpopulation. Regarding post-operative radiation for microscopic residual disease, few data are available, but they are also encouraging, with regard to local control in 3/3 (MGH), 4/6 (UCSF), and 3/3 from another series. (Buffalo) [60], for a total of 10/12 (83%) controlled.

Evaluation of dose delivered relative to control suggests that doses of greater than 5000 cGys are necessary for control of gross disease [57, 98, 59]. It is unclear whether higher doses are necessary. Although there are 4 reported failures of 19 patients treated with doses between 5000 and 6000 cGy, three of the four were felt to represent geographic misses. There were 16/17 tumors controlled with doses equal to or greater than 6000 cGy. From all series the slow regression of desmoid tumors in response to radiation is emphasized in many cases requiring up to two or more years for complete response. As early as 1928, Ewing [61] observed the slow but definite response of desmoid tumors to radiation. Recent reports documented objective changes in most tumors between 2000 and 2500 Gy, in spite of the prolonged interval needed for complete response.

With careful treatment planning, complications have not been significant. Of particular interest are several reported cases [57] in which extremely low dose per fraction radiation was utilized (125–140 cGy) with long term control. This may result in even greater sparing of normal tissues.

In summary, the available data suggests that wide local excision is the appropriate treatment for desmoid tumors when feasible. However, in circumstances of inoperable tumors, recurrent tumors, partially resectable tumors, or tumors resectable only with mutilating surgery, radiation should be considered. Unlike most true sarcomas, desmoids appear to be controlled by radiation alone even in the presence of bulky disease. In cases where surgical removal has been incomplete, radiation has been successful in preventing local recurrence.

The role of radiation therapy in the treatment of true low grade soft tissue sarcomas has been controversial. As described above, surgical excision and postoperative radiation therapy compares favorably with more aggressive surgical procedures in high grade sarcomas. Review of published results for treatment of low grade sarcomas is confusing. The exact surgical techniques are rarely defined, and one suspect that frequently as less aggressive procedure was performed than had the lesion been high grade. Evaluating the true risk of local recurrence after aggressive surgery is therefore difficult.

There is agreement that overall local control and survival is significantly better in grade I sarcomas than higher grade tumors. Data from the American Joint Committee Task Force for Soft Tissue Sarcomas [41] reported 5 year survivals for patients with Stage I tumors as 75%; stage II, 55%; stage III, 29%; and stage IV, 7%.

Similar data have been reported from USCF [26]. However, unlike benign soft tissue tumors, grade I sarcomas are capable of metastasizing, in a small but finite number of cases, and local recurrence may decrease ultimate survival. Therefore, although in tumors such as desmoids, one might be willing to observe the patient after an excision with a questionable margin, a definitive curative approach should probably be undertaken in all true sarcomas.

Surgical reviews do not always separately analyze low grade tumors apart from the high grade sarcomas. Available data from Memorial Sloan Kettering Cancer Center [28] report the frequency of local recurrences after monobloc soft part resection in low grade tumors (G_1) as 25% (8/32) in tumors less than 5 cm and 39% (7/18) in tumors greater than 5 cm. Markhede [24] reports a recurrence in 1/12 low grade tumors; Leibel [26], 6/10 (simple excision only performed in some); Enneking, 0/9 (wide or radical excision); and the NCI [62], 1/12 (same operative excision as for high grade tumors). Because of the wide variation in these data concerning local control rates in low grade sarcomas, it is difficult to establish a policy concerning the addition of radiation therapy in these patients. Some data are available on the use of postoperative radiation therapy in low grade sarcomas. From the MGH [63], local control was achieved after complete resection and postoperative radiation in 4/4 tumors less than 5 cm and 10/10 greater than 5 cm. Memorial Sloan Kettering Cancer Center [64] reported local control in 12/12 less than 5 cm and 11/11 greater than 5 cm; MDAH, 30/32 less than 5 cm, 11/13, 5 – 8 cm; and 16/18 greater than 8 cm; and NCI series [62], 16/17.

It appears, therefore, that surgery and radiation therapy are very successful when used in combination in low grade sarcomas. However, wide local excision, with preservation of function, may well be equally effective in preventing local recurrence. A randomized study comparing surgery versus surgery and postoperative radiation therapy for low grade sarcoma is presently being carried out at the NCI. Hopefully the results from this study will aide in establishing the role of radiation therapy in low grade soft tissue tumors.

Conclusion

Research is ongoing in numerous centers in Europe and the United States to determine the optimal integration of surgery, radiation therapy, and chemotherapy in soft tissue sarcomas. In high grade extremity soft tissue sarcomas, studies are underway to determine the best method for combining radiation with surgery (i.e., postoperatively, preoperatively, and/or intraoperatively). In addition, the NCI is conducting a randomized study (i.e., surgery alone versus surgery plus radiation) in low grade soft tissue sarcomas of the extremities to determine if adjuvant radiation is necessary.

In retroperitoneal sarcomas, centers are looking at the role of external radiation combined with intraoperative radiation to improve local control. Conclusive results of these studies should be available within the next few years. Unfortunately, distant metastases continue to be the key problem with retroperitoneal sarcomas.

Head and neck and truncal soft tissue sarcomas are uncommon. However, the treatment approach of wide local excision combined with either preoperative or postoperative irradiation should be used if possible to obtain good local control with the least morbidity.

For benign soft tissue sarcomas such as desmoids, the role of radiation therapy is more controversial. However, for inoperable tumors, recurrent tumors, partially resected tumors, or tumors resectable only with mutilating surgery, radiation should be strongly considred.

References

1. Windeyer, S. B., Dische, S. and Mansfield, C. M. The place of radiotherapy in the management of fibrosarcoma of the soft tissues. Clin. Radiol. 17: 32 – 40, 1966.
2. Scanlon, P. W. Split-dose radiotherapy for radioresistant bone and soft tissue sarcoma: Ten years experience. Am. J. Roentgenol. 114: 544 – 552, 1972.
3. McNeer, C. P., Cantin, J., Chu, F. and Nickson, J. J. Effectiveness of radiation therapy in the

management of sarcoma of the soft tissue. Cancer 22: 391 – 397, 1968.

4. Perry, H. and Chu, F. C. H. Radiation therapy in the palliative management of soft tissue sarcomas. Cancer 13: 179 – 183, 1968.

5. Murphy, W. T. Radiation therapy, 2nd edition. W. B. Saunders, Philadelphia, 1967.

6. Cade, S. S. Soft tissue tumors: Their nature history and treatment. Proc. R. Soc. Med. 19: 19 – 36, 1951.

7. Lindberg, R. D., Martin, R. G. and Romsdahl, M. M. Surgery and post operative radiotherapy in the treatment of soft tissue sarcomas in adults. Am. J. Roentgenol. 123: 123 – 129, 1976.

8. Lindberg, R. D., Martin, R. G., Romsdahl, M. M. and Barkley, H. T. Conservative surgery and post operative radiotherapy in 300 adults with soft tissue sarcomas. Cancer 47: 2931 – 2397, 1981.

.9 Rosenberg, S. A. and Glatstein, E. J. Perspectives on the role of surgery and radiation therapy in the treatment of soft tissue sarcomas of the extremities. Sem. Oncol. 8: 190 – 200, 1981.

10. Suit, H. D. Patterns of failure after treatment of sarcoma of soft tissue by radical surgery or by conservative surgery and radiation. Cancer Treatment Synposia 2: 241 – 246, 1983.

11. Carabell, S. C. and Goodman, R. Radiation therapy for soft tissue sarcoma. Sem. Oncol. VIII: 201 – 206, 1981.

12. Potter, D. A., Glenn, J., Kinsella, T., Glatstein, E., Lack, E. E., Restrepo, C., White, D. E., Seipp, C. A., Wesley, R. and Rosenberg, S. A. Patterns of recurrence in patients with high-grade soft-tissue sarcoma. J. Clin. Onc. 3: 353 – 366, 1985.

13. Suit, H. D., Proppe, K. H., Mankin, H. J. and Woods, W. C. Preoperative radiation therapy for sarcoma of soft tissue. Cancer 47: 2269 – 2274, 1981.

14. Wood, W. C., Suit, H. D., Mankin, H. J., Cohen, A. M. and Proppe, K. Radiation and conservative surgery in the treatment of soft tissue sarcoma. Am. J. Surg. 147: 537 – 541, 1984.

15. Shiu, M. H., Turnbull, A. D., Nori, D., Hajdu, S., Hilaris, B. Control of locally advanced extremity soft tissue sarcoma by function saving resection and brachy therapy. Cancer 53: 1385 – 1392, 1984.

16. Sindelar, W. F. and Kinsella, T. J. Intraoperative Radiotherapy: The National Cancer Institute Experience. In Progress in Radio-Oncology, Volume III, Karshor, H., editor, Raven Press, New York (in press), 1986.

17. Eilber, F. R., Mirra, J. J., Grant, T. T., Weisenburger, T. and Morton, D. L. Is amputation necessary for sarcomas? A seven year experience with limb salvage. Ann. Surg. 192: 431 – 438, 1980.

18. Tepper, J. E. and Suit, H. D. Radiation therapy alone for sarcoma of soft tissue. Cancer 56: 475 – 479, 1985.

19. Russo, A., Mitchell, J., Kinsella, T., Morstyn, G. and Glatstein, E. Determinants of radiosensitivity. Sem. Oncol. XII: 332 – 349, 1985.

20. Enneking, W. F., Spanier, S. S. and Malawer, M. M. The effect of the anatomic setting on the results of surgical procedures for soft parts sarcoma of the thigh. Cancer 47: 1005 – 1022, 1981.

21. Leibel, S. A. Soft tissue sarcomas: Therepeutic results and rationale for conservative surgery and radiation therapy. Radiation Oncology Annual 1983, edited by T. L. Phillips and D. A. Pistanmaa. Raven Press, New York.

22. Cantin, J., McNeer, G. P., Chu, F. C., et al. The problem of local recurrence after treatment of soft tissue sarcoma. Ann. Surg. 168: 47 – 53, 1968.

23. Gerner, R. E., Moore, G. E., Pickran, J. W. Soft tissue sarcomas. Ann. Surg. 181: 803 – 808, 1975.

24. Markhede, G., Angervall, L. and Stener, B. A multivariate analysis of the prognosis after surgical treatment of malignant soft-tissue tumors. Cancer 49: 1721 – 1733, 1982.

25. Martin, R. G., Butler, J. J. and Alloss-Saavedra, J. Soft tissue tumors: Surgical treatment and results. In: Tumors of bone and soft tissue, edited by M. D. Anderson Hospital and Tumor Institute, pp. 333 – 347. Year Book Medical 1968, Chicago.

26. Leibel, S. A., Transbaugh, R. F., Wara, W. M., et al. Soft tissue sarcomas of the extremities. Survival pattern of failure with conservative surgery and postoperative irradiation compared to surgery alone. Cancer 50: 1076 – 1083, 1982.
27. Potter, D. A., Kinsella, T., Glatstein, E., Rosenberg, S. A., et al. High grade soft tissue sarcomas of the extremities. Cancer, 1986 (in press).
28. Shiu, M. H. and Hajdu, S. E. Management of soft tissue sarcoma of the extremities. Semin. Oncol.. 8: 172 – 179, 1981.
29. Simon, M. A. and Enneking, W. F. The management of soft tissue sarcomas of the extremities. J. Bone Joint Surg. 48A: 317 – 327, 1976.
30. Suit, H. D., Mankin, H. J., Wood, W. C., et al. Preoperative, intra-operative, and postoperative radiation in the treatment of primary soft tissue sarcoma. Cancer 55: 2659 – 2667, 1985.
31. Rosenberg, S. A., Tepper, J., Glatstein, E., et al. The treatment of soft-tissue sarcomas of the extremities. Prospective randomized evaluations of (1) limb sparing surgery plus radiation therapy compared with amputation and (2) the role of adjuvant chemotherapy. Ann. Surg. 196: 305 – 315, 1982.
32. Tepper, J. E. and Suit, H. D. Radiation therapy of soft tissue sarcomas. Cancer 55: 2273 – 2277, 1985.
33. Fraas, B. A., Tepper, J. E., Glatstein, E., et al. Clinical use of a match-line wedge for adjacent megavoltage radiation field matching. Int. J. Radiation Oncol. Biol. Phys. 9: 623 – 628, 1983.
34. Tepper, J., Rosenberg, S. A., Glatstein, E. Radiation therapy technique in soft tissue sarcomas of the extremity: Policies of treatment at the National Cancer Institute. Int. J. Radiat. Oncol. Biol. Phys. 8: 263 – 273, 1982.
35. Mettlin, C., Priore, R., Rao, U., et al. Results of the national soft-tissue sarcoma registry. J. Surg. Onc. 1982; 19: 224 – 227.
36. Glenn, J., Sindelar, W. F., Kinsella, K., Glatstein, E., Rosenberg, S. A. et al. Results of multimodality therapy of resectable soft tissue sarcomas of the retroperitoneum. Sarcomas of the retroperitoneum. Surgery 97: 316 – 325, 1985.
37. Cody, H. S., III, Turnbull, A. D., Fortnar, J. G., et al. The continuing challenge of retroperitoneal sarcomas. Cancer 47: 2147 – 2152, 1981.
38. Tepper, J. E., Suit, H. D., Wood, W. C., et al. Radiation therapy of retroperitoneal soft tissue sarcomas. Int. J. Radiation Oncology Biol. Phys. 10: 825 – 830, 1984.
39. Stout, A. P. and Lattes, R. Tumors of the soft tissue, In Atlas of Tumor Pathology, 2nd series. Washington, D.C. Armed Forces Institute of Pathology, 1967.
40. Enzinger, F. M. and Weiss, S. W. Soft tissue tumors. St. Louis, C. V., Mosby, 1983.
41. Russell, W. O., Cohen, J., Enzinger, F., Hajdu, S. I., Heise, H., Martin, R. G., Meissner, W., Miller, W. T., Schmitz, R. L. and Suit, H. D. A clinical and pathological staging system for soft tissue sarcomas. Cancer 40: 1562 – 1570, 1977.
42. Costa, J., Wesley, R. A., Glatstein, E. and Rosenberg, S. A. The grading of soft tissue sarcomas. Results of a clinicohistopathologic correlation in a series of 163 cases. Cancer 53: 530 – 541, 1984.
43. Trojani, M., Contesso, G., Loindre, J. M., Rouesse, J., Bui, N. B., deMascarel, A., Goussot, J. F., David, M., Bonichon, F. and Lagarde, C. Soft tissue sarcomas of adults. Study of pathological prognostic variables and definition of a histopathological grading system. Int. J. Cancer 33: 37 – 42, 1984.
44. Sears, H. F., Hopson, R., Inouye, W., Rizzo, T. and Grotzinger, P. J. Analysis of staging and management of patients with sarcomas. A ten year experience. Ann. Surg. 191: 488 – 493, 1980.
45. Suit, H. D., Russell, W. O. and Martin, R. G. Sarcoma of soft tissue: Clinical and histopathologic parameters and response to treatment. Cancer 35: 1478 – 1483, 1975.
46. Van der Werf-Messing, B. and Van Unnik, J. A. M. Fibrosarcoma of the soft tissues. Cancer 18: 1113 – 1123, 1965.

47. Myhre-Jensen, O. A conservative 7 year series of 1331 benign soft tissue tumors. Clinicopathologic data comparison with sarcoma. Acta. Orthop. Scand. 52: 287–293, 1981.
48. Musgrove, J. E. and McDonald, J. R. Extra-abdominal desmoid tumors: A differential diagnosis and treatment. Arch. Pathol. 45: 513–540, 1948.
49. Das Gupta, T. K., Brasfield, R. D. and O'Hara, J. Extra-abdominal desmoids. Ann. Surg. 170: 109–121, 1969.
50. Brasfield, R. D. and Das Gupta, T. K. Desmoid tumors of the anterior abdominal wall. Surgery 65: 241–246, 1969.
51. Benninghoff, D. and Robbins, R. The nature and treatment of desmoid tumors. Am. J. Roentgenol. Rad. Therap. Nucl. Med. 91: 132–137, 1964.
52. Dahn, I., Jonsson, N. and Lundh, G. Desmoid tumors, a series of 33 cases. Acta. Chir. Scand. 126: 309–314, 1963.
53. Reitamo, J. J. The desmoid tumor: IV Choice of treatment, results, and complications. Ach. Surg. 118: 1318–1322, 1983.
54. Enzinger, F. M. and Shiraki, M. Muscula-sphoheurotic fibromatosis of the shoulder girdle (extra-abdominal desmoid): Analysis of thirty cases followed up for ten or more years. Cancer 20: 1131–1140, 1967.
55. Masson, J. K. and Soule, E. H. Desmoid tumors of the head and neck. Am. J. Surg. 112: 615–622, 1966.
56. Hunt, R. T. N., Morga, J. C. and Ackerman, L. Principles in the management of extra-abdominal desmoids. Cancer 13: 825–836, 1960.
57. Greenberg, H. M., Goebel, R., Weichselbaum, R. R., Greenberger, J. S., Chaffey, J. T. and Cassady, J. Radiation therapy in the treatment of aggressive fibromatoses. Int. J. Rad. Onc. Biol. Phys. 7: 309–310, 1981.
58. Leibel, S. A., Wara, W. M., Hill, D. R., Bovill, E. G., DeLorimier, A. A., Beckstead, J. H. and Phillips, T. L. Desmoid tumors: Local control and patterns of relapse following radiation therapy. Int. J. Rad. Onc. Biol. Phys. 9: 1167–1171, 1983.
59. Kiel, K. D. and Suit, H. D. Radiation therapy in the treatment of aggressive fibromatoses (Desmoid tumors). Cancer 54: 2051–2055, 1984.
60. Khorsand, J. and Karakousis, C. P. Desmoid tumors and their management. The American Journal of Surgery 149: 215–218, 1985.
61. Ewing, J. Neoplastic Disease Philadelphia: W. B. Saunders Co., 1928.
62. Glenn, J., Potter, D., Kinsella, T., Glatstein, E. and Rosenberg, S. A. The treatment of low-grade (grade 1) soft-tissue sarcomas and other locally invasive soft-tissue tumors with low metastatic potential. Unpublished data.
63. Shiu, M. H., Castro, E. B., Hajdu, S. I. and Fortner, J. G. Surgical treatment of 297 soft tissue sarcomas of the lower extremity. Ann. Surg. 182: 597–602, 1976.

6. Chemotherapy in advanced soft tissue sarcomas

J. Verweij and H. M. Pinedo

Introduction

Although surgery still constitutes the basic treatment modality of soft tissue sarcomas, we have to consider that the local recurrence rate following surgery alone, was as high as 40–80% [1], while most relapses occur within 3 years [2]. The introduction of postoperative high-dose radiotherapy has reduced this local recurrence rate in extremity lesions [3–6], but still distant metastases wil occur in a major number of these patients. Moreover, because soft tissue sarcomas necessitate high doses of irradiation for effective treatment, this precludes adequate application of this technique in truncal lesions. Metastases of soft tissue sarcomas mainly develop by hematogeneous spreading, while their first site of appearance will frequently be the lungs. The frequent development of metastatic disease has stimulated the use of chemotherapy since the identification of doxorubicin (DX) as an active drug in the early seventies [7]. Later, DTIC and more recently Ifosfamide (IFX) have been identified as active drugs for the treatment of soft tissue sarcomas [8]. A complete remission can only be achieved in a limited number of patients, but there are indications that some of them may be cured [9]. This again stimulates the search for new active drugs. From previous studies it appeared that stratification for histologic subtypes and performance score would offer a more proper evaluation of the results of clinical trials, but unfortunately stratifications of such trials seems hardly feasible [10].

This chapter will review the state of the art in the chemotherapy of advanced soft tissue sarcomas.

Single agent chemotherapy (Table 1)

Doxorubicin (DX) was introduced into clinical trial in 1972 [7], and since then has been identified as the most active single agent in the treatment of soft tissue sarcomas. It has been given to thousands of patients, and in over a 1000 non-pretreated

Pinedo, H. M., Verweij, J (eds) Clinical Management of Soft Tissue Sarcomas
© *1986 Martinus Nijhoff Publishers, Boston. ISBN 0-89838-808-2. Printed in The Netherlands.*

patients a cumulative response rate of 23% was found [11]. Preliminary results in an EORTC study also indicate activity of the drug in pretreated patients, while retreatment with the drug after a good remission on previous DX treatment also sometimes may be effective [12].

The drug appears to have a dose-response relationship for this tumor type, with doses of 60 mg/m^2 or more giving higher response rates than doses of 50 mg/m^2 or less [1, 13], in treatment schedules using the single large dose every 3 – 4 weeks. These intermittent high dose administrations are generally assumed to be the most effective, but they limit our possibilities to combine DX with other my-elosuppressive drugs and additionally face us with the problem of cardiotoxicity. These limitations have stimulated studies on alternative scheduling of DX and re-search on less cardiotoxic anthracycline analogues. In a recent study weekly ad-ministration of 15 mg/m^2 appeared to be equally active but less toxic than ad-ministration of 70 mg/m^2 every 3 weeks [14]. However, this is not a consistent finding, because others found comparable myelosuppression in both methods of administration [15, 16]. Another alternative approach may be the continuous in-fusion of DX, which is thought to be less cardiotoxic. However, both presently reported studies also applied concomitant DTIC. The combination achieved a 54% response rate in 50 patients [17, 18], which is equal to similar regimen using single large dose DX (see Table 4). Several anthracycline analogues have been studied, but these will be discussed in Chapter 9, as will be the recent studies on the apparent second best drug in the treatment of soft tissue sarcomas: Ifosfa-mide.

The only other commonly used drug with some activity as a single agent is DTIC (Dimethyl Trianzeno Immidazole Carboxamide). In a single trial in 53 pa-tients a 17% response rate was achieved [19]. However, shortly after this observa-tion, another study indicated the increased response rate of the combination of DX and DTIC as compared with either one of these two drugs alone [20], for which reason no further studies on the single agent activity of DTIC in soft tissue sarcomas have been performed.

Contrasting the data on childhood sarcomas, there are only very limited data on the single agent activity of vincristine (VCR) and actinomycin (DACT) in sar-comas in adults. Only a few responses have been reported. An EORTC study com-

Table 1. Soft tissue sarcomas: active single agents*.

Drug	No. of evaluated patients	Response rate (%)
Doxorubicin	1010	23
Ifosfamide	155	40
DTIC	53	17

* Cumulative data.

paring ifosfamide with cyclophosphamide (CTX) will be discussed in Chapter 10.

Although initial studies on both methotrexate (MTX) [21] and cisplatin (CDDP) [22] suggested some activity in soft tissue sarcomas, additional trials on these drugs indicated that they should be considered inactive [23–28], with the possible exception of mixed mesodermal uterine sarcomas. In this subtype CDDP achieves an 18% response rate [29].

In other previous phase 2 studies insignificant activity has been reported of AMSA, anguidine, 5-azacytidine, Baker's antifol, CCNU, chlorozotocin, cycloleucine, cytembena, DCNU, dianhydrogalactilol, dibromodulcitol, diglycaldehyde, gallium nitrate, hexamethylmelamine, ICRF-159, maytansine, methyl-CCNU, metoprine, PALA, piperazindione, prednimustine, pyrazofurin, vindesine, VM-26 and VP-16-213 [8, 10, 17]. Additional, more recent phase 2 studies will be discussed in Chapter 9.

Combination chemotherapy

In 1971, the Southwest Oncology Group (SWOG) initiated a study, utilizing DX 60 mg/m^2 on day 1 and DTIC 250 mg/m^2/d on days 1–5, repeated every 3 weeks. This regimen is known as ADIC [20]. Because of a response rate of 35%, ADIC has also been studied by other groups with comparable results, achieving 30–47% responses with 4–14% complete remissions [1, 14, 20, 30, 31, 32]. Because of these results, ADIC has become the basis for many other combinations used in soft tissue sarcomas. With sequential additions of VCR and CTX the most commonly used CYVADIC regimen was developed, achieving a 27–53% response rate with 7–18% complete remissions [33–38] (Table 2). The only randomized study including CYVADIC was reported by Pinedo et al. [38] and compared CYVADIC (CTX 500 mg/m^2 i.v., day 1, VCR 1.5 mg/m^2, day 1, DX 50 mg/m^2 day 1, and DTIC 250 mg/m^2/d, days 1–5) with a schedule alternating VCR/CTX and ADIC in similar doses as used with CYVADIC, at 4-week intervals. With CYVADIC 17% complete responses (CR) and 21% partial responses (PR) were achieved, while in the cycling arm a significantly lower response rate

Table 2. Soft tissue sarcomas: various schedules of DTIC infusion in CYVADIC combination chemotherapy.

DTIC (days of treatment)	No. of evaluated patients	Response rate (%)			Ref.
		CR	PR	Overall	
1–5	294	16	27	43	34,37,38
1–3	23	13	39	52	33
1	9	11	0	11	43

84

of 5% CR and 9% PR was achieved (p = 0.001), reflecting the lower activity of CTX/VCR as compared with ADIC. Besides, Dalley et al. [39], using DX/CTX alternating with DACT/DTIC, had similar results. These studies (Table 3) suggest that patients with soft tissue sarcomas do not benefit from alternating non-cross resistant combinations of the currently known drugs. Moreover, the EORTC results [38] indicate that DX should be given 3 or 4-weekly instead of 8-weekly.

Several groups have studied modifications of the CYVADIC regimen in clinical trials (Table 4). The combination of CTX/VCR/MTX/DX (CYOMAD) resulted in a response rate of 27%, which is similar to the results of single agent DX treatment, while CYOMAD appeared to be very toxic [40]. The combination of DX/DTIC and CTX achieved a cumulative response rate of 30% in 115 patients [32, 41], while using the same three drugs but applying continuous infusion infusion of DX and DTIC a 54% response rate was achieved in 50 nonpretreated patients [18].

Trying to reduce the duration of nausea and vomiting, two groups applied DTIC in a high single dose in ADIC [42] and CYVADIC [43] combinations. The results on toxicity were contradictory but, more important, response rates dropped compared to the original schedules (Table 2).

The addition of VDS, CTX and CDDP to ADIC resulted in a 51% response rate in 57 patients [44], but these results have to be confirmed by other study groups, in particular because the added drugs itself are probably inactive as single agents in the treatment of soft tissue sarcomas.

Combinations of DX/DACT [45] DX/DTIC/VCR [20] DX/DTIC/DACT [32] DX/CTX/VCR [46] DX/CTX/VDS [47] DX/CTX/MTX [48, 49] DX/VCR/MTX/DACT [50] DX/VCR/MTX/DACT/DTIC/CLB [50] DX/Me-CCNU [51] or VCR/DACT/CTX [46] did not show advantage over single agent therapy with DX or combination chemotherapy with ADIC or CYVADIC, either because of worse response rates, or because of increased toxicity. These data suggest, that CTX, VCR and DACT are inactive agents in soft tissue sarcomas in adults, although in the CYVADIC regimen CTX and VCR appear to add something to the effect of ADIC.

From all studies it is indicated, that the time to achieve a response may vary

Table 3. Soft tissue sarcomas: alternating combination chemotherapy regimen.

Drugs	No. of evaluated patients	Response rate (%)			Ref.
		CR	PR	Overall	
DX/DTIC alt. CTX/VCR	78	5	9	14	38
DX/CTX alt. DACT/DTIC	20	0	20	20	39
DX/DTIC/VCR/MTX alt. DX/DTIC/CTX	34	12	15	27	40

widely and be very prolonged, reflecting the slow regression of soft tissue sarcomas.

In combination chemotherapy, the advantage of CYVADIC over ADIC may be found in the higher number of complete responses achieved with CYVADIC. In particular those patients achieving a complete response may benefit from chemotherapy, as Yap [9] reported 21% of them to have a disease-free survival of 5 years or more. Although follow-up is somewhat shorter, the EORTC study appears to confirm these results [38]. This indicates that a small number of patients with advanced soft tissue sarcomas may potentially be cured with chemotherapy. Moreover, several studies have indicated that in general complete responders experience a survival benefit over partial- or non-responders [9, 21, 36, 38]. Related to this topic is the important observation, within the EORTC study [38], that the response rate was much higher in patients with a good performance score (PS). In fact, PS was the most important prognostic factor, which may explain some of the controversion in reported response rates. Again this stresses the necessity of stratification for PS in future studies on soft tissue sarcomas. Other prognostic factors related with a high incidence of response and a long survival are female sex, weight loss of less than 5% and age less than 60 years [32, 38, 51], besides size of the tumor and histologic grade. The observation that old patients appear

Table 4. Soft tissue sarcomas: combination chemotherapy regimen other than CYVADIC*.

Drugs	No. of evaluated patients	Response rate (%)			Reference
		CR	PR	Overall	
DX/DACT	22	10	18	28	45
DX/DTIC°	442	11	25	36	14,20,32,42
DX/DTIC/CTX°	165	13	30	43	18,32,41
DX/DTIC/CTX/VDS/CDDP	57	12	39	51	44
DX/DTIC/VCR	80	10	40	50	20
DX/DTIC/DACT	92	9	15	24	32
DX/CTX/VCR	62	3	16	19	46
DX/CTX/VDS	31	26	22	48	47
DX/CTX/MTX	188	–	–	20	48
DX/CTX/MTX	41	4	34	38	49
DX/CTX/MTX/AMPB	46	0	10	10	49
DX/VCR/MTX/DACT	34	–	–	44	50
DX/VGR/MTX/DACT/DTIC/CLB	33	–	–	27	50
DX/Me-CCNU	41	7	42	49	51
DX/Me-CCNU/VCR	42	–	–	26	50
VCR/CTX/DACT	57	2	9	11	46

* Only series with more than 20 patients.
° Cumulative data.

to be less responsive, is probably related to the necessity of dose reduction as well as their generally poorer PS [38].

In conclusion, the number of active drugs currently available for the treatment of soft tissue sarcomas, is still limited to three: doxorubicin, ifosfamide and DTIC. In combination chemotherapy two regimen, ADIC and CYVADIC, appear to be superior over the others, while CYVADIC results in a higher number of complete responses than ADIC. This may be important because a small number of patients achieving a complete response may potentially be cured. It seems obvious, that future studies will have to focus on the development of new drugs.

References

1. Pinedo H. M. and Kenis Y. (1977): Chemotherapy of advanced soft tissue sarcomas in adults. Cancer Treat. Rev. 4: 67 – 86.
2. Lindberg R. D., Martin R. G. and Ramsdahl M. M. (1975): Surgery and postoperative radiotherapy in the treatment of soft tissue sarcomas in adults. Am. J. Roentgen. Rad. Ther. Nucl. Med. 123: 123 – 129.
3. Gerson R., Shiu M. H. and Hajdu S. I. (1982): Sarcoma of the buttock: A trend toward limb-salvage resection. J. Surg. Oncol. 19: 238 – 242.
4. Leibel S. A., Tranbaugh R. F., Wara W. M., et al. (1982): Soft tissue sarcomas of the extremities. Survival and patterns of failure with conservative surgery and postoperative irradiation compared to surgery alone. Cancer 50: 1076 – 1083.
5. Rosenberg S. A., Suit H. D., Baker L. H. and Rosen G. (1982): Sarcomas of the soft tissue and bone. In: Cancer (DeVita V. T., Hellman S. and Rosenberg S. A., eds.), pp. 1036 – 1093, J. P. Lippincott, Philadelphia.
6. Abbatucci J. S., Bowlier M., de Ranieri J., et al. (1983): Conservative treatment of soft tissue sarcomas: Long term results in 69 cases. Proc. ECCO 2: 137.
7. Bonadonna G., Beretta G., Tancini G., et al. (1975): Adriamycin (NSC-123127) studies at the Istituto Nazionale Tumori, Milan. Cancer Chemother. Rep. 6: 231 – 245.
8. Verwey J. and Pinedo H. M. (1985): Randomized trials in soft tissue sarcomas in adults. In: Randomized Trials in Cancer: A critical review by sites (Stevin M. L. and Staquet M. J., eds.), Raven Press, New York (in press).
9. Yap B. S., Sinkovics J. G., Burgess M. A., et al. (1983): The curability of advanced soft tissue sarcomas in adults with chemotherapy. Proc. ASCO 2: 239.
10. Verweij J. and Pinedo H. M. (1985): Clinical trials in adult soft tissue sarcomas. In: Clinical Trials in Cancer Medicine (Bonadonna G. and Veronesi U., eds.), pp. 317 – 334, Academic Press, New York.
11. Verweij J., van Oosterom A. T. and Pinedo H. M. (1985): Melanomas, soft tissue and bone sarcomas. Eur. J. Cancer Clin. Oncol. (in press).
12. Legha S., Benjamin R., Mackay B., et al. (1981): Reutilization of adriamycin in previously treated patients. Proc. ASCO 22: 534.
13. O'Bryan R. M., Luce J. K. and Talley R. W. (1973): Phase II evaluation of adriamycin in human neoplasma. Cancer 32: 1 – 8.
14. Borden E. C., Amato D., Enterline H. T., et al. (1983): Randomized comparison of adriamycin regimens for treatment of metastatic soft tissue sarcomas. Proc. ASCO 2: 231.
15. Mitts D. L., Gerhardt H., Armstrong D., et al. (1979): Chemotherapy for advanced soft tissue sarcomas. Results of phase I and II cooperative studies. Texas Medicine 75: 43 – 47.

16. Chlebowski R. T., Paroly W. S. and Pugh R. P. (1980): Adriamycin given as a weekly schedule without a loading course: Clinically effective with reduced incidence of cardiotoxicity. Cancer Treat. Rep. 64: 49 – 51.

17. Stewart D. J., Benjamin R. S. and Baker L. (1979): In: Therapeutic progress in ovarian cancer, testicular cancer and the sarcomas (van Oosterom A. T., Muggia F. M. and Cleton F. J., eds.) pp. 453 – 479, Martinus Nijhoff, The Hague.

18. Benjamin R. S. and Yap B. S. (1983): Infusion chemotheraphy for soft tissue sarcomas. In: Soft tissue sarcomas (Baker L. H., ed.) pp. 109 – 116, Martinus Nijhoff, Boston.

19. Gottlieb J. A., Benjamin R. S., Baker L. H., et al. (1976): Role of DTIC (NSC-45338) in the chemotherapy of sarcomas. Cancer Treat. Rep. 60: 199 – 203.

20. Gottlieb J. A., Baker L. H. and O'Bryan R. M. (1975): Adriamycin (NSC-123127) used alone and in combination for soft tissue sarcomas. Cancer Chemother. Rep. 6: 271 – 282.

21. Subramanian S. and Wiltshaw E. (1978): Chemotherapy of sarcoma. A comparison of three regimens. Lancet I: 683 – 687.

22. Karakousis C. P., Holtermann D. A. and Holycke E.D. (1979): Cis-di-chlorodiammine platinum (II) in metastatic soft tissue sarcomas. Cancer Treat. Rep. 63: 2071.

23. Buesa J. M., Mouridsen H. T., Santoro A., et al. (1984): Treatment of advanced soft tissue sarcomas with low-dose methotrexate: a phase II trial by the EORTC soft tissue and bone sarcoma group. Cancer Treat. Rep. 68: 683 – 684.

24. Isacoff W. H., Eilber F., Tabbarah H., et al. (1978): A phase II clinical trial with high-dose methotrexate therapy and leucovorin rescue. Cancer Treat. Rep. 62: 1295.

25. Karakousis C. P., Rao U. and Carlson M. (1980): High dose methotrexate as secondary chemotherapy in metastatic soft tissue sarcomas. Cancer 46: 1345.

26. Samson M. K., Baker L. H., Benjamin R. S., et al. (1979): Cis-dichlorodiammine platinum (II) in advanced soft tissue and bone sarcomas: a Southwest Oncology Group study. Cancer Treat. Rep. 61: 2027.

27. Bramwell V. H. C., Brugarolas A. and Mouridsen H. T. (1979): EORTC phase II study of cisplatin in CYVADIC-resistant soft tissue sarcoma. Eur. J. Cancer. Clin. Oncol. 15: 1511 – 1513.

28. Brenner J., Magill G. B., Sordillo P., et al. (1982): Phase II trial of cisplatin (CDDP) in previously treated patients with advanced soft tissue sarcomas. Cancer 50: 2031.

29. Thighpen T., Singleton H., Homesley H., et al. (1982): Phase II trial of cis-diamminechloroplatinum (DDP) in treatment of advance or recurrent mixed mesodermal sarcoma of the uterus. Proc. ASCO 1: 110.

30. Beretta G., Bonadonna G., Bajetta E., et al. (1976): Combination chemotherapy with DTIC (NSC-45388) in advanced malignant melanoma, soft tissue sarcomas and Hodgkin's disease. Cancer Treat. Rep. 60: 205 – 211.

31. Omura G. A., Major F. J., Blessing J. A., et al. (1983): A randomized study of adriamycin with and without dimethyl triazenoimmidazole carboxamide in advanced uterine sarcomes. Cancer 52: 626 – 632.

32. Pazdur R. and Baker L. M. (1985): Treatment of advanced soft tissue sarcomas. In: Management of soft tissue and bone sarcomas (van Unnik J. A. M., van Oosterom A. T. and Pinedo H. M., eds.), Raven Press, New York (in press).

33. Bui B., Chavergue J., Durand M. and Brunet R. (1981): Chimiothérapie palliative des sarcomas des tissus mous de l'adults par une association cyclophosphamide-vincristine-adriamycin-dacarbazin (CYVADIC). Bull. Cancer 68: 1 – 5.

34. Karakousis C. P., Rao U. and Park H. C. (1982): Combination chemotherapy (CYVADIC) in metastatic soft tissue sarcomas. Eur. J. Cancer. Clin. Oncol. 18: 33 – 36.

35. Pfeffer M. R., Silke A. and Biran S. (1983): Modified CYVADIC for soft tissue sarcomas. Proc. ECCO 2: 133.

36. Yap B. S., Baker L. H., Sinkovics J. G., et al. (1980): Cyclophosphamide, vincristine, adriamy-

cin and DTIC (CYVADIC) combination chemotherapy for the treatment of advanced sarcomas. Cancer Treat. Rep. 64: 93 – 98.

37. Yap B. S., Burgess M. A., Sinkovics J. G., et al. (1981): A 5-year experience with cyclophosphamide, vincristine, adriamycin and DTIC (CYVADIC) chemotherapy in 169 adults with soft tissue sarcomas. Proc. ASCO 22: 534.

38. Pinedo H. M., Bramwell V. H. C., Mouridsen H. T., et al. (1984): CYVADIC in advanced soft tissue sarcoma: A randomized study comparing two schedules. Cancer 53: 1825 – 1832.

39. Dalley D. M., Levi J. A., Nesbitt R. A. (1981): Cyclical combination chemotherapeutic regimen in adult soft tissue sarcoma. Cancer Clin. Trials 4: 163 – 165.

40. Lynch G., Magill G. B., Sordillo P. and Golbey R. B. (1982): Combination chemotherapy of advanced sarcomas in adults with CYOMAD(S7). Cancer 50: 1724 – 1727.

41. Blum R. H., Corson J. M., Wilson R. E., et al. (1980): Successful treatment of metastatic sarcomas with cyclophosphamide, adriamycin and DTIC (CAD). Cancer 46: 1722.

42. Saiki J. H., Rivkin S. W., Baker L. H., et al. (1982): Adriamycin and single dose DTIC in soft tissue and bone sarcomas. A Southwest Oncology Group study. Proc. ASCO 1: 181.

43. Bernard S. A., Capizzi S. A., Rudnick S. A., et al. (1982): A one-day combination chemotherapy (CYVADIC) regimen in soft tissue sarcomas. Proc. ASCO 1: 170.

44. Spielman M., Le Chevalier T., Sevin D., et al. (1984): Association doxorubicine, vindesine, cyclophosphamide, DTIC and cisplatin (DCAVC) in soft tissue sarcomas. Cancer Chemother. Pharm. (Suppl.) 14: 60.

45. Brenner D. E., Chang P. and Wiernik P. H. (1981): Doxorubicin and dactinomycin therapy for advanced sarcomas. Cancer Treat. Rep. 65: 231 – 236.

46. Schoenfeld D. A., Rosenbaum Ch., Horton J., et al. (1982): A comparison of adriamycin versus vincristine and adriamycin and cyclophosphamide, versus vincristine, actinomycin D and cyclophosphamide. Cancer 50: 2757 – 2762.

47. Brenner J., Magill G. B., Wissel P., et al. (1983): Chemotherapy of patients with advanced soft tissue sarcoma with use of DVA (Vindesine sulfate), adriamycin and cyclophosphamide (DAC). Cancer 52: 1142 – 1145.

48. Presant C. A., Lowenbraun S., Bartolucci A. A. and Smalley R. V. (1981): Metastatic sarcomas: Chemotherapy with adriamycin, cyclophosphamide and methotrexate, alternating with actinomycin D, DTIC and vincristine. Cancer 47: 457 – 465.

49. Presant C. A., Bartolucci A. A., Lowenbraun S., et al. (1984): Effects of amphotericin B on combination chemotherapy of metastatic sarcomas. Cancer 53: 214 – 218.

50. Magill G. B., Golbey R. B. and Krakoff I. H. (1977): Chemotherapy combinations in adult sarcomas. Proc. ASCO 19: 332.

51. Rivkin S. E., Gottkes J. A., Tighpen T., et al. (1980): Methyl CCNU and adriamycin for patients with metastatic sarcomas. Cancer 46: 446 – 451.

7. Adjuvant chemotherapy for soft tissue sarcomas

Vivien H. C. Bramwell

Introduction

Many aspects of the management of adult soft tissue sarcoma remain controversial. Although surgical removal is the core of local treatment, the importance of eradicating all viable tumor must be balanced against a desire to maintain function. Adjuvant radiation therapy may permit more conservative surgery, but the relative merits of pre- and post-operative therapy are still debated. The contribution of other modalities to local control is not resolved.

Even with good local control metastases occur in 30–50% of cases [1–4]. The role of adjuvant chemotherapy in preventing dissemination (and possibly improving local control) has become one of the most controversial issues.

It is hardly surprising that there have been few randomized trials of adjuvant chemotherapy, and most of those that have been reported have major flaws. Soft tissue sarcomas are rare [1, 2], and although the peak age incidence is the 5th and 6th decades, a significant minority will present in the 7th and 8th decades − a group which is unlikely to tolerate aggressive adjuvant therapy. Total macroscopic removal (an eligibility criterion for most adjuvant studies) may not be possible either because of site or bulk of tumor in a further cohort of patients. In addition soft tissue sarcomas present to many disciplines − surgeons in many subspecialties such as orthopedics, head and neck, neurosurgery, cardiothoracic, gynecology and urology − and it may take time to establish referral patterns for clinical trials. In addition, protocols evaluating adjuvant chemotherapy must take account of the particular problems associated with surgery and radiotherapy at particular disease sites.

Even for a common solid tumor such as breast cancer, which has been the object of numerous randomized controlled trials, encorporating thousands of patients, the precise role of adjuvant chemotherapy has been difficult to establish. Even in the group deriving most benefit (premenopausal patients) the difference in overall survival (10–20%) have been modest [5, 6, 7]. Improvements in overall management of soft tissue sarcomas both at initial presentation and by salvage

Pinedo, H. M., Verweij, J (eds) Clinical Management of Soft Tissue Sarcomas
© *1986 Martinus Nijhoff Publishers, Boston. ISBN 0-89838-808-2. Printed in The Netherlands.*

surgery for local and distant relapse have lengthened the median survival, and may ultimately be associated with a higher rate of cure. In specialist centres 70–80% of patients treated without adjuvant chemotherapy may be expected to survive 5 years [8, 9, 10, 11] and thus in this heterogeneous group of tumors with many prognostic variables, known or unknown, large numbers of patients are required to assess the value of adjuvant chemotherapy with a reasonable degree of confidence. In addition, in some instances chemotherapy may delay metastasis, and an adequate duration of follow-up is essential before interpreting the results of any study.

Important prognostic factors include tumor site, size, histological type and grade, local recurrence and adequacy of local treatment. Three aspects of tumor site must be considered. Firstly, the body localization: extremity tumors, particularly distal lesions, do better than centrally located sarcomas such as those in the head and neck and retroperitoneum. However tumor size and adequacy of surgical resection are confounding factors. Superficial versus deep (to fascia) and intracompartmental versus extracompartmental locations have been considered sufficiently important to be included in staging systems proposed by Hadju [12] and Enneking [13] respectively. It has not been firmly established whether particular histological subtypes of sarcoma respond well to chemotherapy [14–16], and this may well reflect the difficulties that even experienced pathologists have in determining cell type. Many tumors show no or minimal features of differentiation at the light microscopic level, and often material is inadequate for electron microscopy or immunochemistry. Although when information is available on histological grade, this has usually been shown to be one of the most important prognostic factors, the criteria for assigning grade are not yet uniformly accepted. Several different systems for grading soft tissue sarcomas have been proposed [4, 17, 18] but results depend heavily on the adequacy of pathological material, whether the slides assessed are representative of the whole material (and many tumors show marked heterogeneity) and the experience, patience and thoroughness of the pathologist. Data are conflicting on the influence of local recurrence on survival. Although an adverse effect was reported by Cantin et al. [3], in a more recent series Edmonson et al. [9] could not establish a detrimental effect. If local recurrence does adversely influence survival, then the adequacy of local treatment will be important in trials of adjuvant chemotherapy, and will in any event influence comparisons of disease free survival.

In such a rare tumor type, accrual of large numbers of patients is possible only in multicentre trials, and even then may take many years. The disadvantages of this approach include variability of management in individual centres, a higher incidence of ineligible/inevaluable patients, more protocol deviations/violations/missing data and delay in collecting data. If the study period is prolonged, future developments may invalidate the central question and interest and accrual may fall off. Nevertheless, these disadvantages are probably outweighed by the benefits of high patient numbers.

In this paper, only those studies which compare a group receiving adjuvant chemotherapy with a concurrent randomized control group receiving no chemotherapy will be considered. The importance of this in the field of sarcomas has been demonstrated by Antman et al. [19] who reported that concurrent, but non-randomized controls eligible for a trial of adjuvant Adriamycin did significantly worse than control patients entered in the randomized study. Also, Rosenberg et al. [20] reported that patients in the control arm of their randomized study had a significantly higher survival than a historical control group of patients who did not receive chemotherapy. This could not be explained by an analysis of known prognostic factors.

Randomized trials of adjuvant chemotherapy

M. D. Anderson

This study reported by Lindberg et al. [21] using adjuvant Vincristine/Doxorubicin/Cyclophosphamide/Actinomycin D was discussed in detail in volume 1 of this series, and no new data have been published. Briefly, 47 patients with trunk and extremity tumors entered the study and at 18 months the disease free and overall survivals for control and chemotherapy groups were 83% and 85% versus 76% and 68% respectively. Thus, after a short follow-up period no benefit was established for this type of adjuvant chemotherapy.

The most important criticisms of this study as discussed by Rosenberg are the small number of patients, short follow-up and heterogeneity of the patient population.

The remaining studies discussed in this chapter have been reported or updated since volume 1 and unless specifically stated otherwise the following criteria for eligibility were applied.
1) Adult patients with histologically confirmed soft tissue sarcoma, excluding embryonal rhabdomyosarcomas.
2) Absence of metastases, either haematogenous or in regional nodes.
3) No prior radiotherapy or chemotherapy.
4) Adequate hematological, renal and hepatic function.
5) Local recurrence did not exclude patients if other criteria were satisfied.
6) Radical treatment of the primary tumor by surgery +/− radiotherapy. Macroscopic residual disease was not allowed but in some studies microscopically involved margins were permitted if postoperative radiotherapy was given.

92

Table 1. Adjuvant chemotherapy regimes.

NCI (A)

DX 50 mg/m^2 d 1, repeat every 28 d to maximum cumulative dose 500 – 600 mg/m^2.
Escalate by 10 mg/m^2 per course to maximum 70 mg/m^2 based on bone marrow
  tolerance.

CTX 500 mg/m^2 IV d 1, repeat every 28 d.
Escalate by 100 mg/m^2 per course to maximum 700 mg/m^2 based on bone marrow
  tolerance.

At maximum dose of DX change to 6 courses of

MTX 50 mg/kg IV over 6 hrs d 1, repeat every 28 d.
Escalate each course by 50 mg/kg to maximum 250 mg/kg.
Leucovorin 15 mg/m^2 IV 2 hrs after completion MTX and every 6 hrs $\times$ 8.

NCI (B)

DX/CTX as above. 5 cycles only. No Methotrexate.

In both cases chemotherapy given concurrently with XRT.

MAYO

8 Courses of:
VCR 1.2 mg/m^2 IV d 1 + 5
CTX 250 mg/m^2 IV d 1, 3, 5.
DACT 0.325 mg/m^2 IV d 1 – 5
  alternating every 6 wks with
VCR 1.2 mg/m^2 IV d 1 + 5
DX 50 mg/m^2 IV d 3
DTIC 250 mg/m^2 IV d 1 – 5
XRT not given in this study.

EORTC

8 Courses of:
CTX 500 mg/m^2 IV d 1
VCR 1.4 mg/m^2 IV d 1
DX 50 mg/m^2 IV d 1
DTIC 400 mg/m^2 d 1 – 5
at 4 weekly intervals commencing after surgery + / − XRT.

DFCI/MGH

DX 90 mg/m^2 every 3 weeks $\times$ 5.
If pre-op XRT (MGH) − 2 courses given prior to surgery, 3 courses after.
If post-op XRT (DFCI) − 2 courses given between surgery and XRT, and 3 after
  completion XRT.

ECOG

DX 70 mg/m^2 every 3 weeks $\times$ 7.
after completion surgery + / − XRT.

National Cancer Institute (NCI)

As the studies of Rosenberg et al., at the NCI were described in detail in volume 1 of this series, only a brief summary and update [11, 22] of the randomized trials will be presented in this chapter.

Between June 1977 and June 1981, adult patients with sarcomas of the extremities and head and neck and trunk were entered into a prospective randomized trial comparing adjuvant chemotherapy comprising Adriamycin, Doxorubicin (DX), Cyclophosphamide (CTX) and high dose Methotrexate (HD-MTX) (Table 1) with no further treatment. Chemotherapy was started immediately postoperatively and was often given concurrently with radiotherapy.

A subsequent study initiated in July 1981 for extremity sarcomas only compared a 14 month course of the same adjuvant chemotherapy with an abbreviated 5 month course of Adriamycin and Cyclophosphamide only (Table 1), the total doses being half those administered in the previous study.

Patients with grade II or III sarcomas of the following histological subtypes were eligible for those protocols — round cell or pleomorphic liposarcoma, pleomorphic rhabdomyosarcoma, synovial sarcoma, fibrosarcoma, neurofibrosarcoma, leiomyosarcoma, malignant fibrous histiocytoma and undifferentiated sarcoma.

In the first study, significant differences in 5 year actuarial disease free ($p = 0.008$) and overall survival ($p = 0.025$) are evident at a median follow-up of 54 months, in favour of chemotherapy, for patients with extremity sarcomas. There have been 9 recurrences and 5 deaths in the 37 patients in the control group. Unfortunately these benefits were obtained at the expense of a 14% incidence of clinical congestive cardiac failure, and a 52% incidence of abnormal left ventricular ejection fraction in patients who completed a full course of adjuvant chemotherapy.

The second study was initiated on the premise that it might be possible to reduce toxicity but maintain efficacy. The study was closed after accrual of 79 patients with extremity sarcomas, 35 receiving standard chemotherapy and 44 abbreviated treatment. Although there are trends in disease free ($p = 0.18$) and overall survival ($p = 0.11$) favouring the standard chemotherapy, the differences are not significant and median follow-up is short.

In parallel with the first trial in extremity sarcomas, a smaller study (31 patients) compared the 3 drug adjuvant chemotherapy (Table 1) with control in patients with sarcomas of the head, neck, breast and trunk. Although there were differences in actuarial 3 year disease free (77% compared to 49%, $p = 0.075$) and overall survival (68% compared to 58%, $p = 0.38$) in favour of chemotherapy, these differences were not significant. A small subset of 15 patients with retroperitoneal sarcomas analyzed separately, did not appear to benefit from adjuvant chemotherapy, and in some instances there was considerable toxicity associated with the use of DX during radiation therapy.

94

The major criticism of these studies is the small numbers in each trial. Even though there were no major discrepancies in known prognostic factors between compared groups, factors such as tumor size, depth, compartment and local recurrence were not considered. Non-extremity sarcomas did not benefit from the same adjuvant chemotherapy and the validity of separating retroperitoneal sarcomas from the remainder of non-extremity tumors, thus magnifying the effects of chemotherapy, is dubious in the context of such a small number of patients. Nevertheless, these studies now have considerable follow-up and were well conceived and executed. The overall results are excellent, reflecting the benefits of management at a specialist centre.

At present follow-up is insufficient for comment on the study comparing full and abbreviated dose chemotherapy, but it also suffers from the problem of small numbers.

Mayo Clinic (MAYO)

A randomized study performed by the Mayo Clinic [23] compared adjuvant chemotherapy with alternating courses of Vincristine (VCR)/Cyclophosphamide (CTX)/Dactinomycin (DACT) and VCR/Doxorubicin (DX)/Dacarbazine (DTIC) at 6 weekly intervals for one year (Table 1) with a control group who received no initial chemotherapy, although it was offered to patients subsequently if a recurrence was excised.

Between June 1975 and April 1981, 177 patients were eligible for the study but only 61 with localized sarcomas agreed to participate. Patients were treated surgically by wide excision or amputation, but patients receiving pre- or post-operative radiotherapy were excluded. Twenty-four patients in each group had extremity sarcomas, the remainder being trunk or visceral tumors. Malignant fibrous histiocytoma, leiomyosarcoma, synovial sarcoma and liposarcoma were the commonest histological types and 75% of patients had (high) grade tumors. Some delay in the appearance of distant metastases was evident for the group receiving chemotherapy (two-sided log rank, p = 0.15), but there was no delay in local recurrences which appeared in 30% of patients within 5 years after randomization. The 30 patients receiving adjuvant chemotherapy only required 3 thorocotomies (in 3 patients) as salvage treatment for metastases compared with 17 (in 7 patients) in the control group. Surgery for local recurrence was required in 14 and 15 instances repectively.

At a median follow-up of 64.3 months, the estimated survival for all eligible patients was 82% at 5 years, with 54% continuously disease free. Although the group receiving adjuvant chemotherapy did not experience a significant survival advantage (two-sided log rank, p = 0.55), in view of the small study population, the authors stated that the data were also consistent with a doubling in survival duration for the group receiving adjuvant chemotherapy. Although local recurrence was commoner in patients who previously had been treated for locally recurrent tumors, their survival was not significantly different from patients treated for primary disease. There was one toxic death as a result of chemotherapy.

The most important deficiency of this study is the chemotherapy regimen. It has been shown in advanced disease that response is related to the dose and frequency of DX [24] and it is rational to expect similar principles to apply to adjuvant therapy. VCR/DACT/CTX in an inactive combination in advanced sarcoma [25] and DX 60 mg/m^2 every 12 weeks was certainly inadequate. In addition numbers were small and only a small percentage of eligible patients were actually randomized. The reasons for excluding patients receiving radiotherapy are not clear. This study does have the advantage of a long duration of follow-up.

European Organization for Research on Treatment of Cancer (EORTC)

Preliminary data from a European trial, which is still in progress, were presented in December 1984 [26]. This trial, initiated by the European Organization for Research on Treatment of Cancer (EORTC) in 1977 has accrued 326 patients with localized soft tissue sarcomas. All histological subtypes and grades with the exception of borderline/very low grade tumors such as fibromatoses and well differentiated liposarcomas, were included.

All tumors were resected surgically, and although the type of operation was not specified, complete macroscopic removal was mandatory. If microscopic residual disease was present or there was less than one centimeter of healthy tissue around the tumor specimen, postoperative irradiation was given. In addition radiotherapy was required after resection of locally recurrent tumors unless amputation was performed or if a second exploration was required because of inadequate primary excision. The treatment given was the radical technique currently employed by each radiotherapist, but minimum dosages were specified − (50 Gy) in 4 weeks (5 fractions per week) or the biological equivalent (calculated from TDF tables of Orton [27]) for tumors located outside the true pelvis, and (40 Gy) in 4 weeks or biological equivalent for those in the pelvis. Patients had to be fit to start chemotherapy no later than 13 weeks after the first resection of the primary tumor or local recurrence, and randomization was not permitted until radiotherapy, if indicated, had commenced.

Patients were randomized between a chemotherapy arm (eight courses of CYVADIC at 4 weekly intervals (Table 1) and a control arm who received no further treatment but were followed in the same way.

As of October 1984, 326 patients had entered the study. Sixty-six (20%) were considered to be ineligible for the following reasons: − radiotherapy inadequate or not given when required (28 pts), reviewed histology not soft tissue sarcoma (13 pts), missing data (7 pts), advanced disease at entry (7 pts), poor physical condition or age ≥70 yrs (5 pts), inadequate surgery (4 pts), prior chemotherapy

(1 pt), and late randomization (1 pt). There remained 125 eligible patients receiving CYVADIC and 135 controls. On-study data were available for 118 and 129 eligible patients respectively. Limb sarcomas comprised 64% of the total, radiotherapy had been administered postoperatively to 47% of patients and 17% had been treated for locally recurrent tumors. The male to female ratio was 1.22 with a median age of 43 years. Amputation had been performed in 35% of patients with limb sarcomas and microscopic disease at resection margins was noted in 15% of all cases. There was an even distribution of patients, according to these factors, between the two treatment arms. Central histopathological review showed malignant fibrous histiocytoma (24%), liposarcoma (16%) and synovial sarcoma (14%) to be the commonest cell types but 46% of cases remained to be reviewed.

At a mean follow-up time of 119 weeks, 89 (37%), of the 241 eligible patients with follow-up information had relapsed, with 37 experiencing local recurrence, 52 distant metastases and 12 relapsing at both sites. Fifty-one (21%) had died, 43 of malignant disease, 2 due to toxicity (infection and bleeding) and 6 of unrelated causes. Sixty-two patients had completed 8 courses of chemotherapy and 32 remained on treatment. Ten patients relapsed while receiving chemotherapy, 8 refused further treatment, 2 stopped because of intercurrent illness and chemotherapy was terminated in 4 because of myelosuppression. For limb sarcomas, and also for tumors at all sites, significant differences in relapse free and overall survival between the two arms have not emerged and accrual to this study continues.

This study uses the most active drug combination in adult soft tissue sarcomas. It has accrued large numbers of patients, thus compensating for many of the heterogeneities of this patient population. Although the study has been open for 8 years and continues accrual the question remains relevant. Median follow-up is of course short, but detailed survival data according to treatment have not been presented in this preliminary communication. The relatively high rate of ineligibility may be criticized, but additional analysis including all entered patients would eliminate any bias.

As Doxorubicin (DX) is the only drug [24] that is well established as having >20% activity as a single agent in metastatic disease, several groups have elected to study high dose DX alone as adjuvant chemotherapy. The Dana Farber Group based their randomized trial on a small study [28], using matched historical controls, which suggested benefit for this type of adjuvant treatment.

Gynaecologic Oncology Group

In a study from the Gynaecologic Oncology Group [29], patients with stage I and II completely resected uterine sarcomas of all histological types entered a randomized study comparing DX 60 mg/m^2 every 3 weeks for 8 doses, with no further treatment. Pelvic radiotherapy was at the discretion of the investigator, provided the decision was made prior to the chemotherapy randomization. Eligible patients were stratified by stage and prior radiotherapy.

Between 1973–1982, 225 women entered this study of whom 46 (20%) were ineligible and 23 (10%) inevaluable. Seventy-five evaluable patients received DX and 81 were in the control arm. Histological subtypes were leiomyosarcoma − 48 pts; heterogenous mixed mesodermal − 45 pts; homologous mixed mesodermal − 48 pts; endometrial stromal − 12 pts; other − 3 pts. Twenty-five (16%) were stage II, of whom 13 received pelvic radiotherapy.

There was no significant difference in the relapse rate for patients receiving DX: 31/75 (41%)* compared with 43/81 (53%)* in the control group. The duration of progression free interval and median survival (60 months) were not prolonged by DX.

Although pulmonary recurrences were commoner in leiomyosarcoma, and extrapulmonary relapses occurred with mixed mesodermal sarcomas, there was no evidence that adjuvant chemotherapy influenced the incidence or pattern of recurrence in either group.

This study has a large patient population, and focuses on a specific group of sarcomas. There is a reasonable duration of follow-up. The dose of DX could have been more aggressive but is probably adequate. A major flaw is the high rate of ineligibility and inevaluability and no analysis has been made to see if this could have introduced bias.

Dana Farber/Massachusetts General Hospital/Eastern Oncology Group (DFCI/MGH/ECOG)

Antman et al. [30] have reported preliminary results from two independent randomized protocols in soft tissue sarcoma examining the value of adjuvant DX. The total dose of DX, 450–490 mg/m², was similar for both studies, and the regimens are described in Table 1. Visceral sarcomas and lesions with microscopically involved margins were excluded from the ECOG study but were eligible for the DFCI/MGH study. Primary tumors were treated by radical resection (>2 cm margins DFCI/MGH, >5 cm margins ECOG), or conservative surgery (1–2 cm margins, enucleation not permitted) and postoperative irradiation (60–67.5 Gy over 6.5–7 wks in 2 Gy fractions). Some patients at MGH received preoperative radiotherapy, but no further details were given.

The 45 patients entered into the DFCI/MGH study and 33 patients entering the ECOG study were pooled for further analysis. Thirty-eight patients received adjuvant Adriamycin and forty were allocated to the control group. Apart from a preponderence of visceral sarcomas (7 vs 1) in the control group, there was an

___

* Updated figures January 30, 1985, personal communication.

even distribution of patients between the two arms according to disease site and stage, with a total of 47 extremity lesions, 26 head, neck and trunk sarcomas, and 5 retroperitoneal tumors. AJC stages [31] were: IIB − 23 pts; IIIA − 11 pts; IIIB − 36 pts; IVA − 6 pts (2 unknown).

With follow-up ranging from 1−72 months (median 38), twenty-three (29%) patients had died, and there were no significant differences between control and chemotherapy arms for relapse free (p = 0.10) and overall (p = 0.59) survival. This was true for both extremity and non-extremity lesions. Although the shape of the survival curves suggested a delay in the development of metastases in the DX arm there were no significant differences in time to local or distant failure (p = 0.21). The authors commented that in view of the limited patient accrual and short follow-up, the probability of detecting a difference in disease free interval of 20% (60% vs 80%) was 57%, whereas the probability of finding a 15% difference was 39%. Symptomatic cardiomyopathy occurred in 2/38 (5%) of patients receiving DX.

The results of this study are preliminary and even combining results from two slightly different protocols (which may be suspect) the numbers are insufficient. Follow-up is short and the studies remain open to accrual.

University of California (UCLA)

Eilber and associates [10] at University of California, in 1981, initiated a randomized study which compared 5 courses of DX 40 mg/m^2 IV daily × 2 every 4 weeks with a group receiving no further chemotherapy. Treatment of primary tumors during this period was by i.a. DX daily × 3 followed by radiation therapy (3.5 Gy) fractions × 5, and then wide surgical excision.

Results of this study as of January 1985* show 11 recurrences among 50 patients receiving DX and 21 recurrences in the control group of 58 patients. There had been 2 deaths in the DX group and 7 in the control arm. This study continues to accrue patients.

Data from this study are limited, but accrual seems substantial and a full report is awaited with interest.

Conclusions

To summarize, there have been four randomized trials in adult patients with soft tissue sarcomas, which compare adjuvant combination chemotherapy with control. Only one of these [11] has shown significant differences in disease free and overall survival for a subset of patients with extremity tumors. The chemotherapy

* Personal communication.

regimen used was aggressive and was associated with significant cardiotoxicity, and also impairment of fertility [32, 33]. However, only preliminary data are available from another of these trials [26], and the efficacy of adjuvant CYVADIC is sub-judicae. The study from the Majo Clinic [23] demonstrated a non-significant delay in the appearance of distant metastases (although not local recurrences) and operations for removal of pulmonary metastases were less frequent in the chemotherapy group. Approximately 20–30% of such patients may survive 5 years [34, 35] but the rest will experience further relapses, and thus this discrepancy in salvage surgery rate may eventually translate into differences in survival. Nevertheless, in view of the toxicity of adjuvant chemotherapy, delay in metastasis, without overall improvement in survival, is not sufficient to justify its routine use.

Four studies [10, 29, 30] have used varying dose/schedules of adjuvant Doxorubicin and their combined accrual of eligible patients is 342. This therapy does not appear to have benefitted patients with uterine sarcoma and at present there is no clear evidence for improvement in relapse free or overall survival for sarcomas at all sites. However these 3 studies continue to accrue patients, and follow-up is short. In addition, very limited data are available from the UCLA study [10].

Thus one [11] of 8 randomized controlled studies has established benefit for adjuvant chemotherapy, but only in a subset of patients with extremity tumors, and on the basis of a small series of 65 patients. Congestive cardiac failure occurred in 14% of patients receiving chemotherapy. Other studies have found some delay in the appearance of metastases and trends, in favour of chemotherapy, towards improved disease free and overall survival. Four of these studies [10, 26, 30] continue to accrue patients and it is possible that with sufficient numbers of patients and prolonged follow-up, a benefit may be established for adjuvant chemotherapy. Equally, present chemotherapy regimens may not be adequate, and future developments in adjuvant treatment may have to await regimens with improved efficacy in advanced disease, or entirely novel approaches. At present, the conclusion that adjuvant chemotherapy for soft tissue sarcomas should remain within the context of randomized clinical trials (with a no-chemotherapy control group) is inescapable.

References

1. Rosenberg S. A., Suit H. D., Baker L. H., Rosen E., 1982. Sarcomas of the soft tissue and bone. In: Cancer. Principles and Practice of Oncology. DeVita V. T., Hellman S., Rosenberg S. A., eds. J. B. Lippincott Co., Philadelphia, Toronto, 1036–1093.
2. Rosenberg S. A., Glatstein E., 1983. The management of local and regional soft tissue sarcomas. In: Principles of Cancer Treatment. Carter S. K., Glatstein E., Livingston R. B., eds. McGraw-Hill, 697–706.
3. Cantin J., McNeer G. P., Chu F. C., Booher R. J., 1968. The problem of local recurrence of

after treatment of soft tissue sarcoma. Ann. Surg. 168: 47 – 53.

4. Enzinger F. M., Weiss S. W., 1983. Soft tissue tumors. C. V. Mosby.

5. Nissen-Meyer R., Kjellgren K., Mansson B., 1982. Adjuvant chemotherapy in breast cancer. Recent Results in Cancer Research 80: 142 – 148.

6. Rossi A., Bonadonna G., Valagussa P., Veronesi U., 1981. Multimodel treatment in operable breast cancer: five year results of the CMF programme. Br. Med. J. 282: 1427.

7. Fisher B., Redmond C., Wolmark K. N., Wieand H. S., 1981. Disease free survival at intervals during and following completion of adjuvant chemotherapy. The NSABP experience from three breast cancer protocols. Cancer 48: 1273 – 1280.

8. Sordillo P. P., Magill G. B., Shiu M. H., Lesser M., Hadju S. I., Golbey R. B., 1981. Adjuvant chemotherapy of soft-part sarcoma with Alomad (S4). J. Surg. Onc. 18: 345 – 353.

9. Edmonson J. H., 1984. Role of adjuvant chemotherapy in the management of patients with soft tissue sarcomas. Cancer Treat. Rep. 68: 1063 – 1066.

10. Eilber F. R., Guiliano A. E., Huth J., Mirra J., Morton D. L. Limb salvage for high grade sarcomas of the extremity: Experience at the University of California, Los Angeles. Proceedings National Institutes of Health Consensus Development Conference on limb sparing treatment and adjuvant chemotherapy for adult soft tissue and osteogenic sarcomas. Dec. 3 – 5, 1984. Cancer Treat. Symposia 3: 49 – 58, 1985.
tant Advances in Oncology. (In Press.)

12. Hadju S. I., 1979. Pathology of soft tissue tumors. Philadelphia, Lea & Fabiger.

13. Enneking W. F., Spanier S. S., Goodman M. A., 1980. Current concepts review. The surgical staging of musculo-skeletal sarcoma. J. Bone & Joint Surg. 62A: 1027 – 1030.

14. Pinedo H. M., Bramwell V. H. C., Mouridsen H. T., Somers R., et al., 1984. CYVADIC in advanced soft tissue sarcoma: a randomized study comparing two schedules. A study of the EORTC Soft Tissue and Bone Sarcoma Group. Cancer 53: 1825 – 1832.

15. Presant C. A., Lowenbraun S., Bartolucci A. A., Smalley R. V., and the South Eastern Cancer Study Group, 1981. Metastatic sarcomas: chemotherapy with Adriamycin, Cyclophosphamide, and Methotrexate alternating with Actinomycin D, DTIC, and Vincristine. Cancer 47: 457 – 465.

16. Schoenfeld D. A., Rosenbaum C., Horton J., Wolter J. M., Falkson G., Deconti R. C., 1982. A comparison of Adriamycin versus Vincristine and Adriamycin and Cyclophosphamide versus Vincristine, Actinomycin D and Cyclophosphamide for advanced sarcoma. Cancer 50: 2757 – 2762.

17. Costa J., Wesley R. A., Glatstein E., Rosenberg S. A., 1984. The grading of soft tissue sarcomas: results of a clinicohistopathologic correlation in a series of 163 cases. Cancer 53: 530 – 541.

18. Trojani M., Contesso G., Coindre J. M., Rouesse J., et al., 1984. Soft tissue sarcomas of adults: study of pathological prognostic rarities and definition of a histopathological grading system. In: J. Cancer 33: 37 – 42.

19. Antman K., Wood W., Price K., Amato D., Corson J., et al., 1983. A comparison of randomized versus concurrent controls. Proc. Am. Ass. Cancer Res. 23: 146.

20. Rosenberg S. A., Tapper J., Glatstein E., Costa J., Young R., et al., 1983. Prospective randomized evaluation of adjuvant chemotherapy in adults with soft tissue sarcomas of the extremities. Cancer 52: 424 – 434.

21. Lindberg R. D., Murphy U. K., Benjamin R. S., Sinkovics G. G., et al., 1976. Adjuvant chemotherapy in the treatment of primary soft tissue sarcomas: a preliminary report. In: Management of primary bone and soft tissue tumors. Year Book Med. Pub. Chicago, 343 – 352.

22. Rosenberg S. A., Chang A. E., Glatstein E. Adjuvant chemotherapy for the treatment of extremity soft tissue sarcomas: Review of National Cancer Institute experience. Proceedings National Institutes of Health Consensus Development Conference on limb sparing treatment and adjuvant chemotherapy for adult soft tissue and osteogenic sarcomas. Dec. 3 – 5, 1984. Cancer Treat. Symposia 3: 83 – 88, 1985.

23. Edmonson J. H., Fleming T. R., Ivins J. C., Burgert E. O., et al., 1984. Randomized study of

systemic chemotherapy following complete excision of non-osseous sarcomas. J. Clin. Onc. 2: 1390 – 1396.

24. Bramwell V. H. C., Pinedo H. M., 1982. Treatment of soft tissue sarcoma. Proceeding International Symposium on Adriamycin. Hakone, Japan, July 14 – 16.

25. Baker L., Benjamin R., Fine G., Saiki J., Rivkin S., 1979. Combination chemotherapy in the management of disseminated soft tissue sarcomas: a Southwest Oncology Group (SWOG) study. Proc. Am. Soc. Clin. Onc. 20: 378.

26. Bramwell V. H. C., Rouesse J., Santoro A., Buesa J., et al. European experience of adjuvant chemotherapy for soft tissue sarcoma, preliminary report of a randomized trial comparing CYVADIC with control. Proceedings National Institutes of Health Consensus Development Conference on limb sparing treatment and adjuvant chemotherapy for adult soft tissue and osteogenic sarcomas. Dec. 3 – 5, 1984. Cancer Treat. Symposia 3: 99 – 108, 1985.

27. Orton C. G., 1972. Analysis and the time/dose/fractionating problem. AAPM Quarterly Bulletin 6: 173 – 175.

28. Antman K., Blum R., Corson J., Wilson R., et al., 1980. Effective adjuvant chemotherapy for localized soft tissue sarcoma. Proc. Am. Ass. Cancer Res. 21: 141.

29. Omura G. A., Blessing J. A., Lifshitz S., Mangan C., et al. A randomized clinical trial of adjuvant Adriamycin in uterine sarcomas: a Gynaecologic Oncology Group study. J. Clin. Onc. (In Press.)

30. Antman K., Amato D., Lerner H., Suit H., Corson J., et al. Adjuvant Doxorubicin for sarcomas: data from the Eastern Cooperative Oncology Group and Dana-Farber Cancer Institute/Massachusetts General Hospital studies. Proceedings National Institutes of Health Consensus Development Conference on limb sparing treatment and adjuvant chemotherapy for adult soft tissue and osteogenic sarcomas. Dec. 3 – 5, 1984. Cancer Treat. Symposia 3: 109 – 116, 1985.

31. Russell W. O., Cohen J., Enzinger F., Hadju S. I., et al., 1977. A clinical and pathological staging system for soft tissue sarcomas. Cancer 40: 1562 – 1570.

32. Dresdale A., Bonow R. O., Wesley R., Palmeri S. T., et al., 1983. Prospective evaluation of Doxorubicin-induced cardiomyopathy resulting from post-surgical adjuvant treatment of patients with soft tissue sarcomas. Cancer 52: 51 – 60.

33. Shamberger R. C., Sherins R. J., Rosenberg S. A., 1981. The effects of post-operative adjuvant chemotherapy and radiotherapy in testicular function in men undergoing treatment for soft tissue sarcoma. Cancer 47: 2368 – 2374.

34. Flye M. W., 1982. Treatment of metastatic cancer. In: Cancer: Principles and Practice of Oncology. DeVita V. T., Hellman S., Rosenberg S. A., eds. J. B. Lippincott, Philadelphia, 1539 – 1552.

35. Bramwell V. H. C., Pinedo H. M., 1982. Treatment of metastatic bone and soft tissue sarcomas. In: Principles of Cancer Treatment. Carter S. K., Glatstein E., Livingston R. B., eds. McGraw-Hill, 718 – 783.

8. Intra-arterial infusion and perfusion chemotherapy for soft tissue sarcomas of the extremities

Alberto Azzarelli, Leandro Gennari, Maurizio Vaglini, Mario Santinami and Salvatore Andreola

Introduction

Surgery alone was for many years the classic primary treatment for operable soft tissue sarcomas. However, despite accuracy in local resection, most conservative operations and some amputations failed for local recurrence, only in part restrained by complementary radiation therapy [1−3].

In recent years, regional treatments with infusion or perfusion of chemotherapeutic agents have been investigated in many institutions, with promising results. The main task is to achieve a better local control and consequently avoid amputation. The basic rationale of regional chemotherapy of cancer is to deliver a large amount of drug to a selected tumor-bearing area with little systemic toxicity and side effects. These treatments are indicated for inoperable but confined lesions or for limb-sparing strategies for large lesions of the extremities.

In the management of soft tissue sarcomas of limbs and girdles, the main procedures evaluated for delivering regional chemotherapy are continuous infusion of chemotherapy through a catheter placed percutaneously in a selected arterial region, and perfusion of the affected extremity with chemotherapy and hyperthermia combined with extracorporeal circulation (ECC). The theoretical rationale of these therapies is mostly different thus determining different indications and eventual combinations.

The purpose of intra-arterial preoperative infusion is to achieve a clinico-pathologic improvement of the primary lesion, and therefore to adopt a simpler surgical conservative approach. In the meantime, the systemic drug circulation is expected to control or prevent possible micrometastases. Moreover, the surgical specimen will document the chemosensitivity of the treated lesion to the infused drug − useful information to select cases which could benefit from postoperative adjuvant treatment. In contrast, hyperthermic perfusion (HP) chemotherapy by ECC is locally more agressive and is an attempt to cure the lesion even without surgery. However, it does not provide systemic control, and the local pathologic response is possibly documented only by needle sampling.

Pinedo, H. M., Verweij, J (eds) Clinical Management of Soft Tissue Sarcomas
© *1986 Martinus Nijhoff Publishers, Boston. ISBN 0-89838-808-2. Printed in The Netherlands.*

These procedures differ also for the drug-concentration/infusion-time ratio. In fact, intra-arterial infusion is usually a highly diluted solution administered for 24 h a day for several days, whereas perfusion of limbs is a hyperconcentrated solution perfused by ECC for about 1 h.

Intra-arterial infusion chemotherapy

Theoretical rationale

The main purpose of intra-arterial access for chemotherapy is to increase the amount of drug delivered to a tumor: the theoretical expectancy is a more effective local response and less systemic toxicity. Intra-arterial chemotherapy combines two procedures, each effective by itself: intra-arterial administration and slow continuous infusion. The main difference between intra-arterial versus intravenous administration of chemotherapy is that with the former all the delivered drug passes first through the tumor-bearing arterial region. At the first passage a part of the agent will be extracted by and active against the tumor tissue, a second part will be extracted by normal tissue of the same arterial region, and a third part will enter into the systemic circulation: part of this last fraction will be detoxified or eliminated (usually by the liver or kidneys) and part will return to the other body tissues and to the affected area again. With this model, a large amount of the infused drug, if properly selected, should be extracted by the tumor, more than is extracted after intravenous injection. In a mathematical comparison between intravenous and intra-arterial infusion, Chen and Gross [4] stated that doxorubicin (DX), when given intra-arterially to the extremities, should increase its regional level, improve local tumor response, but not reduce systemic toxicity.

Slow intra-arterial infusion versus bolus should increase or at least leave unmodified the drug portion extracted by the tumor, but should allow a better catabolism of the agent, hence reducing toxicity. Continuous infusion could enhance antitumor activity if the drug had a cycle phase-specific activity and a short serum half-time [5]. DX is not a phase-specific antitumoral agent, and its serum half-life is between 10 and 30 h; for these reasons its slow continuous infusion should be protracted for a very long time (100 to 200 h) to achieve an improved therapeutic index. In addition, it has been documented that slow continuous infusion, even if intravenous, results in less cardio- and myelotoxicity [6, 7]. The combination of intra-arterial access and very slow continuous infusion should achieve an increased local effect and decreased systemic toxicity. Experimental studies support this expectancy [8, 9]. Transferring mathematical and experimental models to clinical experience, the main difficulty is to have a quantitative idea of the real entity of the single 'parts' of drug which support the theoretical model.

In fact, many factors are expected to affect the amount of drug delivered to and eventually extracted by the tumor mass: a) the dimension of the bulky tumor in relation to the blood arterial flow in that particular region; b) the grade of vascularization of the lesion; c) the position of the tip of the catheter and the choice of selective cannulation; d) a possible change in blood and drug supply due to frequent angiospasm caused by the catheterization — this complication is much more frequent in small arteries; e) any anatomical or pathological situation which could slow down the hematic return (this factor is thought to facilitate and improve the contact between tumor and drug, therefore some authors have developed new devices and methodologies to obtain an artificial slow down, such as a tourniquet fastened at the limb root, or infusion of chemotherapy plus microspheres causing temporary capillary obstruction, but no significant data have been reported [10−12]); f) the specific sensitivity of the individual lesion to the chosen drug. Most of these factors do not rely on mathematical models or are not easily measurable: because of the influence of these variables, it is difficult to predict on a theoretical basis the local results of limb regional infusion, and only clinical experience will document the reliability of these premises.

The technique

Catheter positioning

Intra-arterial infusion of limbs and girdles is performed through a catheter with the terminal tip located in the artery that irrigates the area where the lesion under treatment is located. In former experiences [13, 14], soft catheters in Teflon or Silastic were preferred and placed intra-arterially by surgical access. The present technique, which is widely accepted, employs firmer catheters of polyethylene, placed percutaneously. The access for the lower extremities is the femoral artery, and for the upper extremities the femoral or brachial artery. The catheter is usually placed at the time of diagnostic angiography, which is feasible, safe and repeatable for almost any location of a sarcoma in the extremities.

The amount of drug dispensed to the lesion depends on the vascular anatomy of the infused region and on the position of the tip of the catheter. Most lesions of the lower limbs are vascularized by branches of the femoral artery, and the tip of the catheter is placed in the external iliac artery (Fig. 1). For lesions of the pelvic girdle, the catheter tip is placed in the common iliac artery or selectively in the internal iliac artery. The homolateral access is indicated for lesions of limbs, and contralateral for lesions of the groin and pelvis. When possible, the drug solution should be injected against blood flow to obtain a better plasma distribution. For the upper extremities, in our experience the homolateral brachial access resulted in frequent local complications mainly due to extravasation or peculiar distribution of the drug in selected small areas of the skin: the femoral access is preferred (Fig. 2).

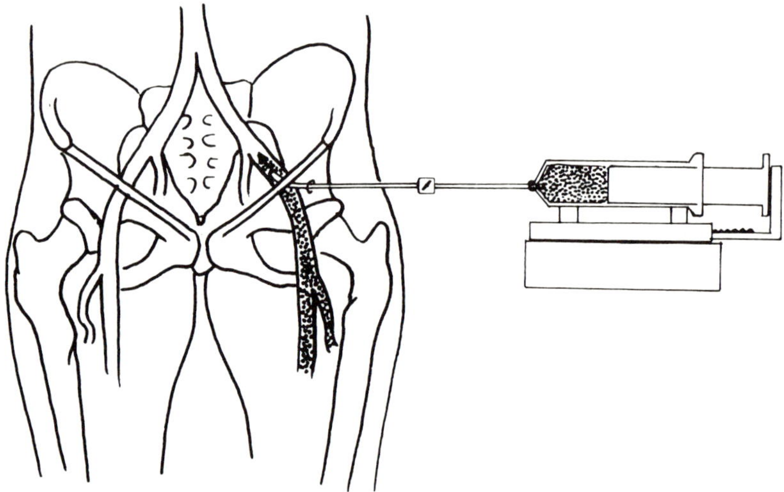

Figure 1. Schematic illustration of the infusional set and typical lodgement of the catheter for intra-arterial infusion of the lower extremities. The tip of the catheter is placed against the blood flow in the external iliac artery. This usual position is appropriate for infusion of the entire limb. Different positions of the catheter tip are indicated when selective arterial supply to the lesion is documented.

The drug

Not all chemotherapeutic agents are suitable for regional treatment. The drug delivered intra-arterially should have: a) specific tropism for the kind of tumor under treatment; b) direct activity without the necessity of metabolic transformation; c) easy clearance from the capillaries towards the interstitial space even at low plasma concentration; d) early catabolism by liver or kidney; e) good stability for several hours at room temperature even when highly diluted.

In the management of soft tissue sarcomas, DX is the drug of first choice, and it is appropriate for intra-arterial delivery according to the aforementioned items. In fact, clinical and experimental studies have confirmed its enhanced tissue concentration, tumor uptake and improved effect by intra-arterial administration [4, 9, 15–17]. Moreover, DX improves tumor cell sensitivity to radiation therapy [18–20]: this peculiarity is the theoretical basis of the protocol outlined at the University of California at Los Angeles (UCLA), where radiation therapy is performed immediately after infusion of DX and before surgery [21]. Using DX in slow infusion to prevent a possible diminished effect, it is important to shield all the infusinal set (syringe, vial, tubing) from daylight and to keep the prepared solution no longer than 12 h.

The infusion

The chosen drug is administered at slow continuous infusion according to the treatment schedule. The constant and precise infusional flow is controlled by an

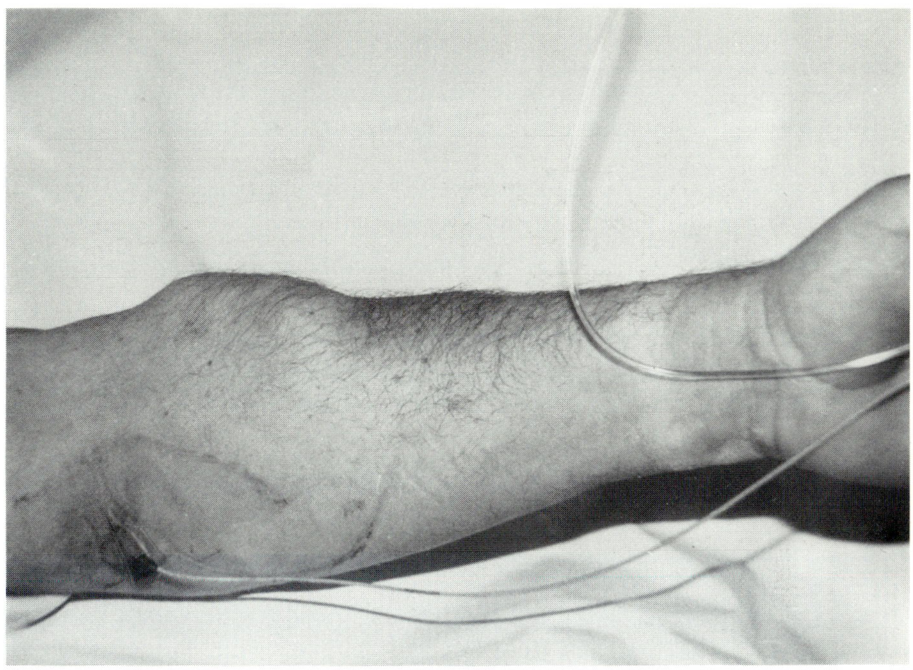

Figure 2. Brachial artery catheterization for infusional treatment of a lesion of the forearm. At the percutaneous access to the artery, a moderate blushing and edema are visible. For this reason the femoral access is now preferred also for infusion of the upper extremity.

external electric pump or other volumetric device suitable for arterial pressure. The patient remains in bed during the therapy: the more common complication during infusion is catheter dislodgement with severe tissue damage due to extravasation. Catheters can be left in place for up to 15 days or more without any complication; if displaced, it can be reinserted immediately or after recovery from a possible hematoma.

Infusional therapy can be repeated many times, at the classic interval of 3–4 weeks. In our experience, a total of 45 catheterizations in 32 cases were performed without complication. In six cases, the catheter was accidently dislodged: in two cases, it was replaced, and in the other four the remaining drug was given intravenously. Catheterization of the brachial artery frequently resulted in mild local side effects such as disappearance of the radial pulse, and temporary and reversible episodes of cyanosis. Two cases developed a typical distribution or extravasation of DX in superficial planes of the anteromedial surface of the mid arm, with edema and pain, which was treated with an ice pack and intradermal or intravenous hydrocortisone; in both cases a second programmed cycle of chemotherapy was repeated intravenously. Local recovery was almost complete after four weeks without necrosis or ulcers. At the end of the cycle, the catheter can

108

be easily removed without any particular attention except for compression of the percutaneous access.

Recent investigations

Intra-arterial infusion of chemotherapeutic agents was first described in detail by Watkins and Sullivan [13] in the sixties, only for inoperable malignancies (mostly carcinomas of the liver or head and neck) treated with 5-fluorouracil or methotrexate. In the same years in our Institute DX was first experienced by intra-arterial infusion for head and neck advanced cancer, with poor results [22, 23]. In 1974, a cooperative study [24] between UCLA and our Institute collected 42 cases of different malignancies treated according to this new approach: besides the substantial discouraging results, the small group of soft tissue sarcomas (six cases) suggested the opportunity of further investigations, which were carried out in later years.

The most important experience in this field was reported by the UCLA group, where a systematic multimodality management or extremity sarcomas has been used since 1975 [21, 25–29]. Detailed data on 100 cases [28] have documented with proper methods and adequate follow-up the role of this multimodal treatment in terms of tumor shrinkage and reduction of cell viability, reducing the number of local recurrences with prevalence of conservative operations versus amputations: among cases treated with limb-salvage surgery, the local recurrence rate was only 3%, and the overall actuarial three-year survival was 64% [27]. An up-to-date preliminary report collected 181 cases and confirmed these data with 97% local control [29]. The pathologic response seemed to be related to the grading of the tumor: grades I and II had a median tumor cell necrosis of about 40%, whereas grade III was about 75% of the bulky tumor. It should be pointed out that this pathologic response is related to both intra-arterial chemotherapy and radiation therapy. In fact, the treatment schedule consists of preoperative intra-arterial DX (60–90 mg, total dose given continuously for 72 h) immediately followed by radiation therapy up to 35 Gy in 10 fractions, then, after a few days, radical surgery. In 1981 the radiation dose was reduced from 35 to 17.5 Gy. Patients treated with this new radiation regimen showed 20% less tumor necrosis, but local control was adequate. Their impression was that DX had a better therapeutic index when given intra-arterially than intravenously, as pharmacokinetic studies suggest. However, this clinical advantage has not yet been proven, and their patients are presently randomized to systemic or intra-arterial preoperative DX administration.

Many other experiences have been reported in the literature, but a comparison of data is difficult due to different selection of cases, various therapeutic regimens, and small number of cases. Krabill et al. [30] in 1977 reported their experiences with intra-arterial DX in 40 advanced cases, including only five sarcomas, without conclusions. Marée et al. [14] in a 14-year period collected 21 cases of advanced sarcomas treated with intra-arterial chemotherapy according to different drug regimens, mostly with methotrexate, and only five with intra-arterial DX in combination (CYVADIC): their experience documented and confirmed the important role of radiation therapy in combination with DX. Intra-

Table 1. Review of recent investigations with detailed information on results and follow-up.

Author (year)	Therapeutic rationale	I.A. drug and dose	No. of cases	Conservative operations	Local recurrence	Metastasis	Metastasis-free interval*	Follow-up of patients*	3-year & DFS[†] (%)	Ref.
Marée (1980)	I.A. CT + RT + SURG	DX (in CYVADIC) I.A. bolus	5	4	–	3	8	32	–	[14]
Karakousis (1980)	I.A. CT + SURG + adjuvant CYVADIC or others	DX 60 mg/m² I.A. bolus	10	5	1	5	5	21	–	[31]
Eilber (1984)	I.A. CT + RT + SURG + adjuvant CT	DX 90 mg total 3-day inf.	100	95	3	–	–	–	64 (61)	[28]
Denton (1984)	I.A. CT + RT + SURG + adjuvant DX + MTX	DX 100 mg total 3-day inf.	20[‡]	20	1	–	–	–	68 (–)	[32]
Mantravadi (1984)	I.A. CT + RT + SURG + adjuvant DX + DTIC	DX 100 mg/m² 10-day inf.	32	29	1	8	6	15	70 (57)	[33]
INT of Milan (1984)	I.A. CT + SURG + eventual RT + eventual adjuvant CT	DX (& DX + CDDP) 100 mg/m² 8-day inf.	32	21	2	12	5	15	55 (53)	

* Median values in months.
[†] In parenthesis, disease-free survival.
[‡] Five with a primary lesion of the trunk, and five with lung metastasis at the time of presentation.
CT, chemotherapy; RT, radiation therapy; inf., infusion; SURG, surgery.

arterial methotrexate plus radiation therapy resulted in complete plus partial clinical remission of the lesion in 9 of 15 cases, with five complete remissions (CR); DX gave clinical remission in five of five, with four CR. Karakousis et al. [31] in 1980 reported 10 cases with operable sarcomas all treated with intra-arterial DX: a good level of gross and histologic postoperative necrosis was achieved; in five cases wide conservative resection was performed, and one recurred. More recently, Denton et al. [32] on 20 cases and Mantravadi et al. [33] on 32 cases employed a regimen similar to that used by UCLA and confirmed the validity of this multimodal approach in terms of limb salvage. Other smaller series or case reports have not provided useful information [15, 34]. Table 1 summarizes the characteristics of major series and our unpublished data.

Experience at the Istituto Nazionale Tumori of Milan

On the basis of reports in the literature and contacts with the group at Los Angeles, in our Institute intra-arterial DX has been delivered to patients with large soft tissue sarcomas of the extremities since 1981 [35, 36]. All selected patients presented a highly malignant primary lesion with the minimal diameter larger than 8 cm and were classified as stage IIb or IIIb according to the system proposed by the American Joint Committee on Staging and End Results [37].

Therapeutic regimens and rationale

Three different schedules of preoperative infusion have been employed in consecutive periods (Table 2), all with intra-arterial DX. The former regimen (scheme A) used intra-arterial DX alone for one preoperative cycle, the second (scheme B) was more aggressive with intra-arterial DX in combination with intra-arterial cis-platinum (CDDP) for two preoperative cycles. Results were not as expected, and the present schedule (scheme C) uses intra-arterial DX alone for two cycles. All the cases were operated on soon after the end of infusion.

Postoperative radiation therapy was indicated when surgical or pathologic judgement of radicality was dubious, or after conservative operations performed on recurrent lesions, but never as palliation after gross intralesional surgery, even if minimal residual disease was left: in this case the patient was reoperated.

Postoperative adjuvant chemotherapy was scheduled in scheme B for responders (pathologic response >50%) with two cycles of i.v. DX (75 mg/m^2) + CDDP (90 mg/m^2) and in scheme C for all cases irrespective of the degree of pathologic response, with i.v. DX (75 mg/m^2) for two dosages.

As of December 1984, 32 patients, have been treated according to this rationale.

Results

A preliminary report of this study has been published on 13 cases [35]. Provisional unpublished data on 32 cases treated according to the three regimens are report-

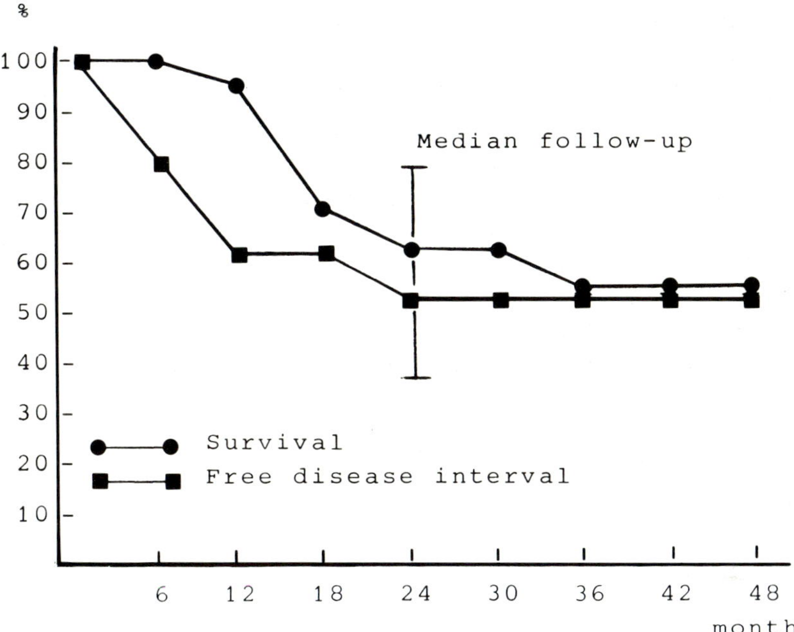

Figure 3. Actuarial survival and disease-free interval of 32 patients treated at the Istituto Nazionale Tumori of Milan with intra-arterial doxorubicin followed by surgery.

ed here (Table 2). The overall results are 21/30 (70%) of pathologic response > 50%, and 2/21 (10%) local recurrence rate after conservative surgery. Long-term results are 55% four-year actuarial survival and 53% four-year disease-free interval (Fig. 3). No local recurrence or metastasis occurred later than 18 months after the primary treatment, and with an overall median follow-up of 24 months the final results can be considered reliable. The role of adjuvant postoperative chemotherapy is not yet evaluable because of the short follow-up of the few patients treated according to schemes B and C, which foresee postoperative treatment.

Tables 3 and 4 report the postinfusional and long-term results stratified by the three chemotherapeutic regimens. Examining the different pathologic responses to the three schemes, the surprising observation is the poor response rate achieved by scheme B (5 responders out of 10) versus scheme A (in 13 of 16). The differences are not significant, but the reason why a more aggressive treatment with intra-arterial DX + CDDP for two cycles did not achieve at least the same results as intra-arterial DX alone for one cycle, also considering that DX was given at the same dose/cycle of $100/m^2$ in both schemes, is not clear. It is unlikely that CDDP, ineffective in the i.v. route [38], could diminish the response to DX. Our impression is that it could depend on the duration of the infusion of DX: eight

112

days for the effective scheme A versus four days in scheme B. This infusion-time-related response rate, if proved, could be an important point in favor of very slow infusion versus bolus, or a few hours of infusion. In theory, tumor cells exposed for a long time to the chosen effective drug, even at low concentration, are expected to be found in a responsive phase, as suggested by Stephens [39]. Moreover, the DX serum half-time of $10-30$ h suggests that continuous infusion shorter than $48-72$ h will not give a detectable improved therapeutic effect.

The histologic results were stratified by histological subtype and grade of vascularization, two parameters which could affect the response rate. According to the major subtypes, in decreasing order, malignant fibrous histiocytoma was responsive in 6 of 7 cases, liposarcoma in 5 of 9 cases, and synovial sarcoma in 1 of 4 (p = 0.1). The degree of vascularity was not predictive for the pathologic response rate, even if some relationship seems to exist within the same subtype (Fig. 4).

It is not easy to state in how many cases the surgical indication was changed

Table 2. Treatment schedules of preoperative intra-arterial chemotherapy employed at the Istituto Nazionale Tumori of Milan, in consecutive periods.

Scheme A

I.A. doxorubicin (100 mg/m²)   SURG

↓ ↓ ↓ ↓ ↓ ↓ ↓ ↓   ↓

1 2 3 4 5 6 7 8   9 – 12

Radiotherapy after dubious radicality or contaminated operations.

Scheme B

I.A. DX (100 mg/m²)	I.A. CDDP (120 mg/m²)	Same schedule		SURG
↓ ↓ ↓ ↓	↓ ↓ ↓ ↓	↓ ↓ ↓ ↓	↓ ↓ ↓ ↓	↓
1 2 3 4	5 6 7 8	22 23 24 25	26 27 28 29	30 – 33

In responders: doxorubicin (75 mg/m² iv) + CDDP (90 mg/m² iv) for 2 postoperative cycles every 21 days. Radiotherapy after any marginal or contaminated operations.

Scheme C

I.A. doxorubicin (100 mg/m²)	Same schedule	SURG
↓ ↓ ↓ ↓ ↓ ↓ ↓ ↓	↓ ↓ ↓ ↓ ↓ ↓ ↓ ↓	↓
1 2 3 4 5 6 7 8	22 23 24 25 26 27 28 29	30 – 33

In all cases: doxorubicin (75 mg/m² iv) for 2 postoperative cycles every 21 days. Radiotherapy after any wide resection, marginal or contaminated operations, and after operations performed on recurrent or residual disease.

Table 3. Clinical and pathologic response to intra-arterial infusion according to three different schemes.

Intra-arterial chemotherapy	No. of clinical improvement	Histologic necrosis > 50%	Histologic necrosis > 90%
Schema A (DX 8-day infusion for 1 cycle)	7/18	13/16	6/16
Scheme B (DX 4-day infusion + CDDP for 2 cycles)	5/10	5/10	3/10
Scheme C (DX 8-day infusion for 2 cycles)	3/ 4	3/ 4	1/ 4
Total	15/32 (47%)	21/30 (70%)	10/30 (33%)

after infusion from amputation to wide resection, but the number of limb-sparing procedures, 21 of 29 operations (72%), is higher than previously performed in our Institute. This data is much more evident if we consider the strict selection of large and invasive primary sarcomas, similar for shape, site and pathologic grading. However, our short-term results after preoperative infusion are not comparable with others because of the higher dose of DX used (100 mg/m^2/cycle), which is almost double that used by Weisenburger et al. [21], and for the histologic documentation of response, which is really related to the use of intra-arterial chemotherapy alone.

Table 4. Long-term results after intra-arterial chemotherapy plus surgery by three different schemes.

Treatment schedule	No. of cases	Lung metastases	Disease-free interval*	No. alive	Overall follow-up*
Schema A (DX alone 1 cycle)	17	9[†]	5	9	39
Scheme B (DX + CDDP 2 cycles)	10	3	8	9	15
Scheme C (DX alone 2 cycles)	4	–	–	4	5
Total	31	12	5	21	24

* Median value in months.
[†] Two cases developed synchronous metastases.

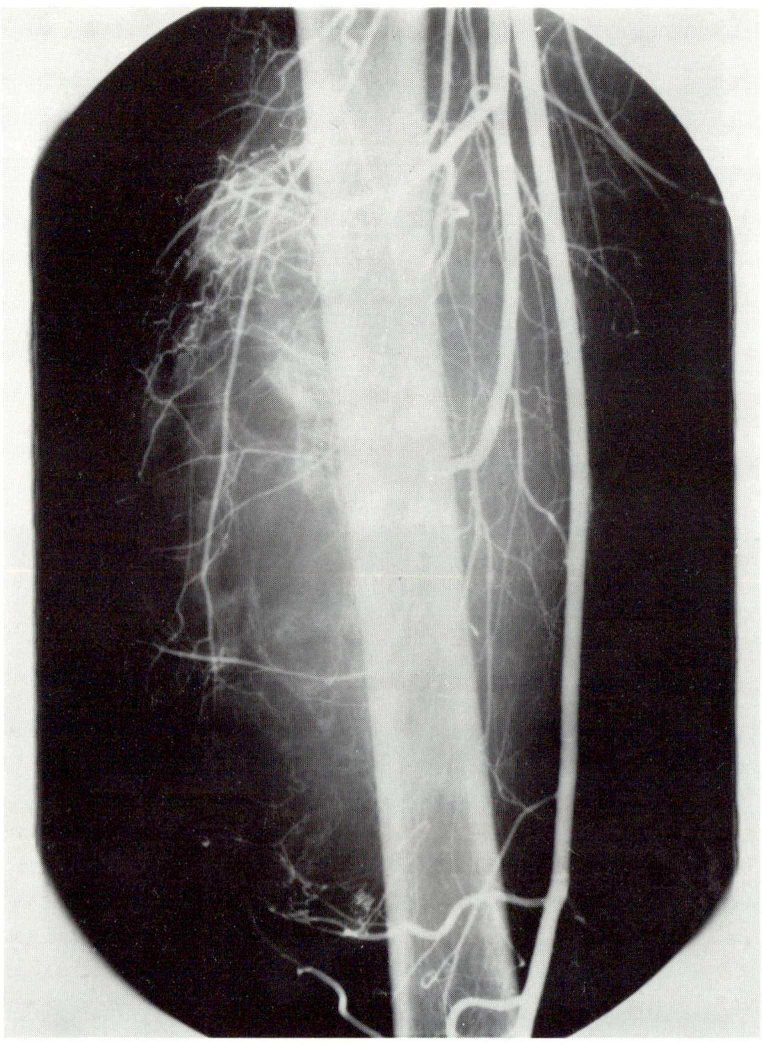

Figure 4. Angiography of a malignant fibrous histiocytoma of the right thigh. The grade of vascularization of the lesion was not predictive of the final result of infusion. This case, with moderate vascularization from the deep femoral artery, showed a histologic postinfusional necrosis of >50%.

Toxicity after preoperative chemotherapy was typical, with complete alopecia in all patients, mild nausea after DX, and more severe nausea and vomiting after DX/CDDP. Mild to severe stomatitis was recorded in four cases. Leukopenia and thrombocytopenia median values were $2\times10^9/l$ and $140\times10^9/l$, respectively, around the 14−15th day after infusion. The wide range of toxicity was peculiar: six cases had a leukopenic nadir below $1\times10^9/l$ and a thrombocytopenia nadir below $40\times10^9/l$, whereas five cases had no toxic effect on hematologic values.

This discrepancy in myelotoxicity was not predictable on the basis of liver and renal function, either before treatment (in fact, all eligible cases had normal hematologic values) or during treatment. Mild impairment of liver function parameters occurred during infusion but did not result in additional toxicity. One death occurred postoperatively for severe systemic sepsis and local infected hemorrhage in the patient who developed the most severe myelosuppression; no other case had relative postinfusional or postoperative complications, and there were no delays in wound healing, irrespective of the degree of leukopenia or thrombocytopenia. Caution is advised in the timing of the operation, which should not be performed when the myelotoxicity nadir is expected (i.e., between the 12th to 16th day after the first day of the last infusion), but immediately after the end of infusion or about a week later. No congestive cardiac failure was recorded, but this complication was also not expected. In fact, the total cumulative dose of DX was only 100 mg/m^2 after scheme A, and 200 mg/m^2 or 350 mg/m^2 after schemes B and C, for patients who received only preoperative infusion or pre- and post-operative chemotherapy, respectively. Moreover, the slow infusion time of DX administration has proved to be less cardiotoxic [7].

Pathologic evaluation of response

The pathologic estimation of the degree of regression is the main objective parameter in short-term evaluation of local response to preoperative chemotherapy. Some difficulties exist when drawing a conclusive pathologic report: a) areas of spontaneous necrosis are not distinguishable from posttreatment necrosis especially in the central portion of the neoplasm, where the former is a common finding. For this reason only foci of necrosis in the peripheral portion of the neoplasm within a mass of viable tumor have been interpreted by some authors as posttreatment regression [26]; b) minor cellular damage (such as hyperchromasia, pyknosis, and cytoplasmic vacuolization) is frequent and should be evaluated in relation to the clinical course. It has little significance per se, because it is difficult to relate such damage to the drug's effect, and to state when cytologic damage is no longer reversible and can be considered at the same level as the necrosis; c) sampling of pathologic tissue is determinant. Histologic examination and estimation of regression should be confirmed in multiple specimens taken from different sites of the tumor; however, peripheral samplings are more significant because recent necrosis is frequently found in peripheral viable portions of the tumor. The possible documented necrosis of the pushing border of the tumor may be a shield against local recurrence, and thus marginal surgery could be considered as adequate.

In our study we followed the definition of Morton et al. [26] were necrosis is 'total absence of identifiable nuclei'; however, when possible we recorded also minor cellular damage. A gross estimation of the percentage of residual viable tumor was recorded and the histologic evaluation was made in 7 – 10 samples of these areas,

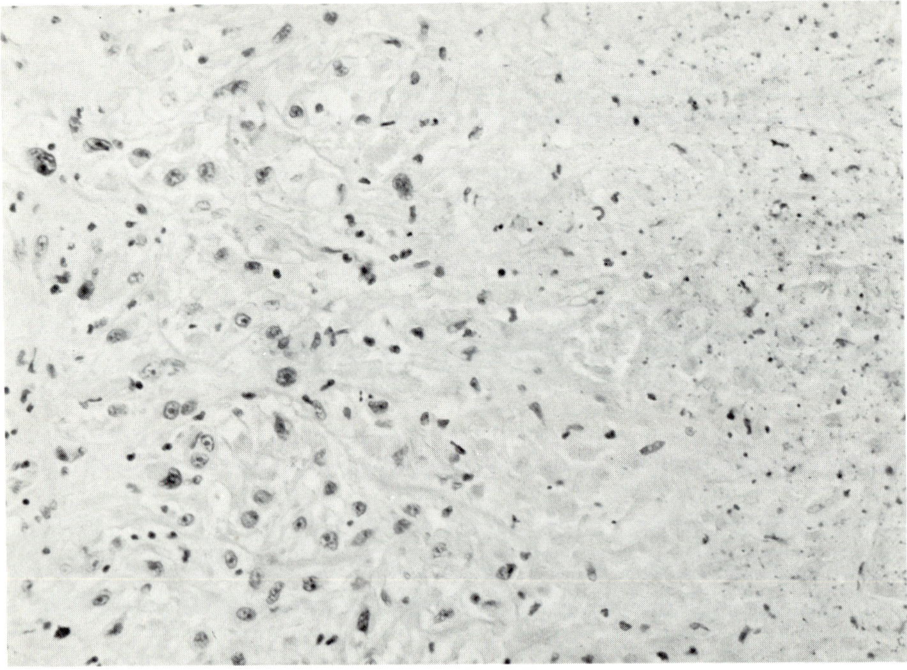

Figure 5. Rhabdomyosarcoma. Postinfusional specimen: small nests of residual tumor cells close to a large area of complete necrosis. (Hem. & Eos., ×400).

especially in the transitional areas with normal tissue surrounding the neoplasm. When possible, the surgical specimen was compared with a preoperative biopsy. The area of complete necrosis was made up of well-demarcated confluent foci of various size, with no cytoplasmic or nuclear structure, and with large deposits of cellular debris and amorphous material (Fig. 5). Significant cytologic changes (hyperchromasia, irregular nuclear shape, cytoplasmic vacuolization) were visible in the transitional zones between the foci of complete necrosis and the residual tumor, whereas in the latter there was no significant cytologic damage. The small- and medium-sized vessels around the tumor did not reveal specific structural changes, and only in rare cases was there evidence of arterial thrombosis. In contrast, in the areas of complete necrosis there were many arterial thrombi, widespread sclerosis of the vascular walls, and occlusion of the lumens. Inflammatory infiltrate was usually scarce. Another peculiar aspect of the tumor regression consisted of large areas of sclerosis where hyalin, dense and acellular fibrous tissue surrounded small nests of residual and morphologically intact neoplastic cells. No definite explanation can be given for this feature, although it may be related to a healing process occurring during the various stages of the treatment (Fig. 6). Excluding two cases which did not reveal any response to chemotherapy, all the others showed a degree of regression ranging from less than 50% to 100%.

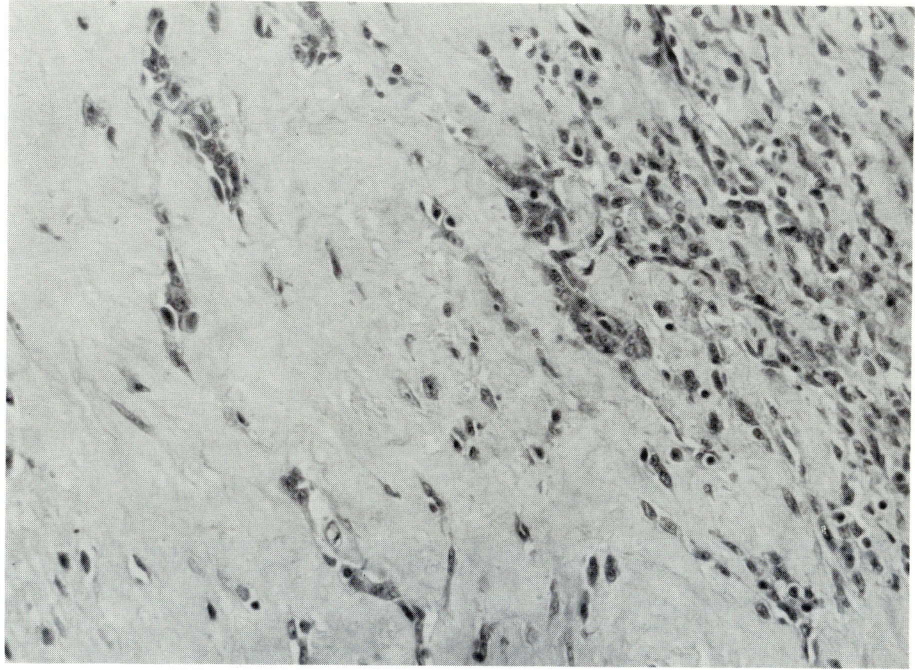

Figure 6. Malignant fibrous histiocytoma. Postinfusional specimen: large area of fibrosis entrapping nests of tumor cells. This fibrosis was not considered as necrosis. (Hem. & Eos., ×250).

Hyperthermic perfusion chemotherapy in extracorporeal circulation

HP chemotherapy by use of ECC is a very new therapeutic method in the treatment of primary and advanced cancer recurrence in the extremities. This method of treatment is based on three basic principles: hyperthermia to which neoplastic cells are more sensitive than normal cells, high drug dose (approximately 10 times more than can be administered by general route), and a synergic action between the hyperthermia and some drugs, resulting in a considerably increased drug action. Two main events occur during ECC: 1) the action of the cytotoxic drug is limited to the diseased extremity; 2) the normal circulation is replaced by ECC, producing a fundamentally new biologic situation in the perfused limb during the treatment.

Theoretical rationale

Considering the biologic aspects and biochemical bases of this method, we should stress that the effect obtained resulted from the combination of two separate factors: a) hyperthermia and b) the intra-arterial administration of high doses of drugs in ECC, resulting in c) induction of a potentiation effect.

Hyperthermia
The use of heat in the treatment of malignancies started more than a hundred years ago, when Busch [40] and Bruns [41] observed tumoral regression after high fever. In 1893, Coley [42] injected bacterial toxins in patients affected by cancers, in order to induce elevated fever for therapeutic use. However, after a period of intense interest, fewer studies on possible applications of heat in cancer therapy were performed. Only in the sixties was there renewed interest in this area, both in experimental and clinical fields. These researchers demonstrated, as first fundamental data, both in vitro and in vivo, a higher sensitivity to heat of tumor cells than normal cells [43−48]. The mechanism of action of temperature is not completely clarified, although a multifactorial action seems probable, modifying physical, biologic and biochemical conditions. Documented targets of the hyperthermic effect are: a) the mitochondria (in fact, many authors have demonstrated a decrease in cellular oxygen consumption after heating [43−45]); b) some functions of the cell membrane concerning the maintenance of electric potential and the control of intracellular pH [43, 49, 50]; c) the synthesis of nucleic acids and proteins, reducing the replication activity of cells, and irreversibly damaging the repair mechanism [45, 51, 52]. Probably, to these effects produced by hyperthermia directly on tumor cells, other effects have to be added: in particular, it seems that hyperthermia can influence the expression of cell surface antigens, so that we may hypothesize a modification of the immunologic response [53]. Even though further studies are needed, numerous experimental and clinical data seem to confirm this hypothesis [48, 54, 55].

Intra-arterial administration with ECC of high dosage drugs
The main advantages of intra-arterial perfusion of an isolated region are: a) maximal drug concentration and regional level, 5−10 times higher than obtainable systemically; b) minimal drug dispersion and systemic leakage with minimal systemic toxicity and immunodeficiency; c) total removal of perfusate and drug from the treated extremity; d) more advantages with regard to the regional administration of heparin for prevention of thrombosis and a possible effect on metastatic development. Conversely, the main limitations are: a) the brief exposure of the cell population to the action of the antitumoral agent; b) the lack of a possible systemic effect of chemotherapy; c) the aggressive surgical approach with possible intra- and postoperative complications, and problems related to ECC.

Synergic effects
Numerous experimental and clinical data indicate a potential effect between hyperthermia and drugs, resulting in an increased cytotoxic activity [51, 56]. This mechanism of action is certainly a complex one and probably different for the

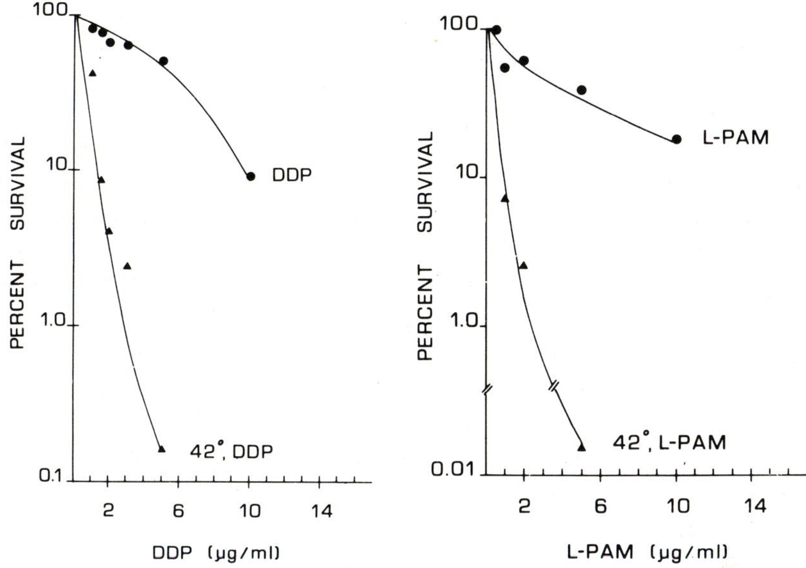

Figure 7. The effect of Cis-platinum and L-PAM enhanced by hyperthermia on melanoma cultured cells.

various drugs. Concerning the two most frequently used drugs in perfusion, L-phenylalanine-mustard (L-PAM) and CDDP, Natali et al. [57], demonstrated the potentiated effect on melanoma (Fig. 7).

Surgical technique

For the lower extremities, perfusion is usually performed through the external iliac vessels, which are reached by the extraperitoneal approach. All tributaries to the external iliac vein are tied. The patient is heparinized (3.3 mg/kg body weight). The internal and external iliac arteries are occluded by tightening umbilical tapes. After arteriotomy and venotomy, catheters are placed into the vascular lumens. Once the catheters are in the proper position, an Esmarch tourniquet is fastened around the base of the extremity in order to achieve complete isolation of the limb. At this point, the catheters are connected to the extracorporeal machine and perfusion is started (Fig. 8). The temperature of the limb is checked frequently by thermistor probes until the desired level is reached (usually 41 °C in the muscle), which generally takes about 30 min. At this time, the cytotoxic drug is given in a single concentrated bolus. Perfusion lasts 60 min from the time of injection of the drug. The muscle temperature is not allowed to go beyond 41 °C. At the end of perfusion, the limb is washed with three liters of saline solution,

120

thus decreasing the temperature of the limb. The heparin action is neutralized with protamine sulfate depending on the clotting time. For upper extremities, the surgical procedure is identical, with the approach via the axillary vessels.

Indications

Until recently, antiblastic HP was performed mainly in the treatment of locally advanced malignant melanoma. The prognosis is always extremely poor for these patients when treated with conventional therapies; five-year survival ranges from 12 to 25%. Isolation perfusion using L-PAM has increased this survival to 54−70% [48]. Concerning the management of soft tissue sarcomas, as already stressed, conservative surgery alone does not provide an adequate local control in many cases. With the same expectancies that encouraged the experiences in intra-arterial infusion, many authors performed HP also for these lesions when located in the extremities.

Recent investigations

In reporting the 30 years experience at the Tulane School of Medicine, Krementz and Muchmore [58] refer to 111 patients with soft tissue sarcomas who were treated by HP alone or HP plus surgery. Several antineoplastic compounds were used in HP but only two cases were treated with DX. It should be noted that DX has not been used in HP because it was documented to precipitate in the presence of a heparin-containing solution [59]. Also, the temperature of the perfusate was modified according to different experiences through the years: after Stehlin's experience published in 1969 [60], Krementz and Muchmore reported that they switched from normothermia to high temperature. The five- and ten-year survival of patients with locally recurrent lesions treated by HP alone or HP plus surgery ranged from 60 to 90%, according to different stratification of the series: the peculiar selection of cases does not provide comparable data. It should be noted that these results are very difficult to interpret also for the difference in histologic types and the variety of postperfusional treatments, i.e., amputation, radiation therapy, intra-arterial chemotherapy with DX, or nothing at all.

Contemporary to this series is that of the M. D. Anderson Hospital as reported by McBride et al. [61]: 110 soft tissue sarcoma patients were treated by HP using L-PAM and actinomycin D alone or in combination. The dosage of the drug was adjusted to each patient, according to the body surface, percent of precalculated leakage to the general circulation, and tissue tolerance (dark skinned individuals were supposed to show a better tolerance); five-year survival in primary sarcomas with a maximum diameter of less and more than 5 cm was 80% and 40%, respectively. No data are reported on survival by histologic subtype because it was not

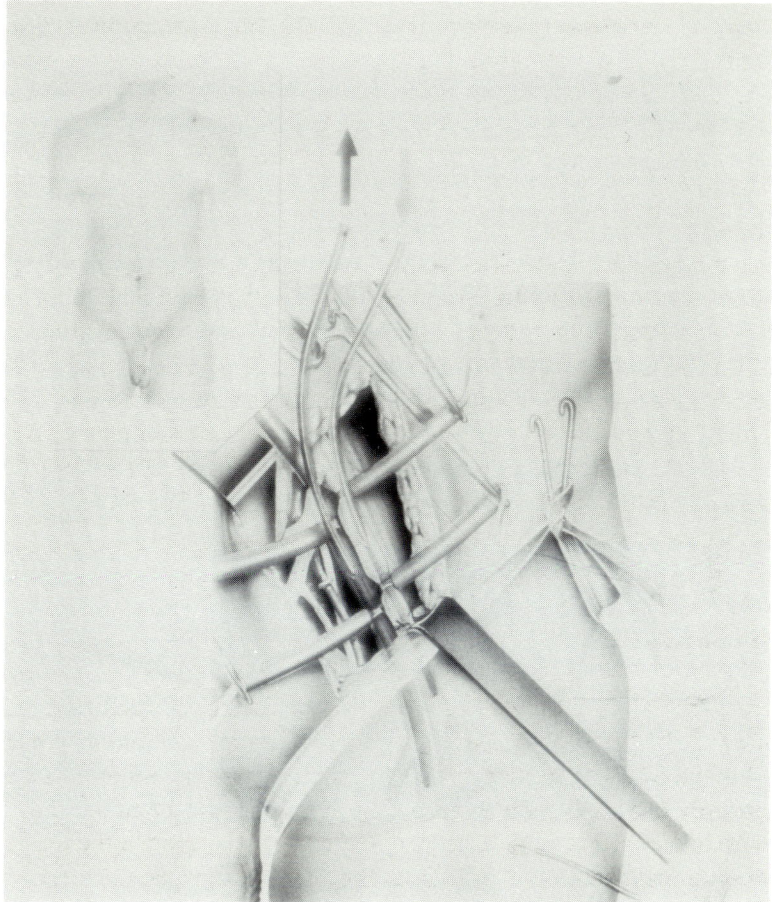

Figure 8. Surgical access to iliac artery and vein for perfusion by extracorporeal circulation.

considered relevant at that time. The five-year incidence of local recurrence and distant metastases was 15% and 18%, respectively. Posttreatment complications depended on the type and number of drugs used and ranged from 11% to 37%.

The same drug schedule was used by Schraffordt Koops et al. [62] in 15 soft tissue sarcoma patients. The temperature ranged from 38°–40°C over 1 h of perfusion. Both histologic type and clinical stage varied widely. The three-year survival in stages I and II, cumulatively considered, was 67%, whereas no stage III patient was alive at one year after treatment. No local recurrences were observed in stages I–IIIA.

Reporting a nonrandomized study on liposarcomas of the limbs, Lehti et al. [63] confirmed that no local recurrences followed HP with L-PAM and actinomycin D, but the mortality rate for distant metastases was higher than 20% at three years of follow-up. Even in this series there was no uniformity of treatment, with 50% of patients submitted to adjuvant therapy and limited surgery. This and the previously reported studies do not show significant improvement with regard to the technique and the results compared to the experience on soft tissue sarcomas of Stehlin et al. [64].

More recently, Braat et al. [65] treated 14 soft tissue sarcoma patients at different stages of disease using HP plus DX plus melphalan. It is noteworthy that this is the first series in which this drug combination was routinely used. DX was added to the perfusate at the dose of 5−40 mg/liter of perfused tissue, associated with melphalan given at 4−25 mg/liter perfused tissue, in some cases limited surgery on the lesion and adjuvant radiation therapy were performed. Five patients underwent amputation due to advanced status of local disease and, in one case, toxicity. Metastasis to distant sites was not hindered by HP, but no local relapses occurred. Nevertheless, it appears difficult to attribute an exact value to results obtained in local control for the wide variety of the doses of drugs administered.

Experience at the INT of Milan

Table 5 reports the results obtained by our team in the treatment of soft tissue sarcomas during the period 1981−1984. Seven patients were perfused with different drugs: L-PAM, actinomycin D, DTIC, CDDP. A histologic response of more than 90% was documented in four of six evaluable cases. Again, the main problem in our series was poor homogeneity in the characteristics of patients and of treatment protocols. We decided to treat these patients on a palliative basis with the hope to avoid demolitive surgery, and these considerations determined the lack of uniformity of treatment.

Thus, we cannot draw any conclusions from these data. However, irrespective of the histologic type and the drug used, an important local response, namely tu-

Table 5. Hyperthermic perfusion for soft tissue sarcomas. Drugs administered and response to treatment at the Istituto Nazionale Tumori of Milan.

Drug	Histologic type	% of tumor necrosis
L-PAM	Liposarcoma myxoid	90
Actinomycin D	Kaposi's sarcoma	90
L-PAM	Clear cell sarcoma	90
DTIC	Clear cell sarcoma	NR
CDDP	Epithelioid sarcoma	90
	Hemangioendothelioma, malignant	NE
	Hemangiopericytoma, malignant	50

NR, no response; NE, not evaluable.

mor necrosis, was obtained, and this was a common achievement in the reported studies. Nevertheless, the role of HP in limb-sparing procedures and the timing in multimodal treatment has still to be defined.

Conclusive considerations

Soft tissue sarcomas are rare tumors. Moreover, many parameters, further stratified in many variables, are involved in the prognostic evaluation: histologic subtype and grade, patient age, site and size of the lesion. In addition, most of the patients come to observation in major institutes after non-successful treatments performed elsewhere.

These features are serious limitations in outlining and evaluating results from any new treatment rationale, selecting homogeneous cases, and thus for programming a controlled study which is not likely to yield reliable data on small series. Convincing suggestions have been reported in the literature, but the real validity of intra-arterial infusion, and even more of HP, is still controversial: they seem to play an important role in performing limb-sparing surgery, but many questions are far from being answered. This survey of studies performed on intra-arterial infusion and isolated perfusion confirms some theoretical expectancies but leaves many questions open.

The role of intra-arterial chemotherapy in performing limb-sparing procedures

Intra-arterial infusion alone may be effective on primary soft tissue sarcoma, but it cannot eradicate the lesion and has to be included in a multimodality management. Recent experiences with multimodality procedures have documented a lower incidence of local recurrence after conservative surgery. Collecting data from the major studies reported in Table 1, only eight local recurrences have been observed after 174 limb-sparing procedures (5%). This number is lower than the recurrence rate after amputation alone: 18% as reported by Cantin et al. in 1968 [1]. However, it is not correct to compare results of recent experiences with historical reviews or past studies reported in the literature, or to relate the present improved data only to sophisticated multimodal strategies. In fact, new proper staging systems, a widely accepted classification of surgical adequacy, and improved surgical techniques and surgical approaches would yield a more effective local control even without ancillary treatments [66, 67]. Only larger series and eventually controlled studies will verify the effective role of preoperative treatment, in practical terms, in limb-sparing procedures.

Intra-arterial versus intravenous preoperative chemotherapy

Experimental and clinical studies have documented that during intra-arterial infusion DX is concentrated more in the tissue of the infused district than systemically, and that after infusion the blood and tissue levels of DX progressively and quickly decrease and assume an identical level between infused and systemic regions [8, 9, 17, 68]. However, it has not been proved clinically that preoperative chemotherapy is more effective when given intra-arterially than intravenously. The group at UCLA is performing a randomized study with intra-arterial versus intravenous DX at the same regimen [29]. In our Institute, in cooperation with our department of experimental oncology, a pharmacokinetic study is underway to evaluate DX levels in blood and tissue samples taken at different times and from different sites (infused versus contralateral limb) from patients treated with intra-arterial DX for sarcomas. Provisional data have documented a higher concentration of DX in venous blood of the affected limb during infusion, and a tumor tissue concentration of the agent from three to six times the normal tissue concentration. This value seems to depend on the time of sampling after infusion: the later this time the higher the difference in DX concentration between tumor and normal tissue. In fact, DX levels decrease more rapidly in normal than in tumor tissue. The difference in DX tissue level between infused versus the contralateral extremity is under investigation.

The role of postoperative adjuvant chemotherapy in responders

When a good histologic local response is documented, is it correct to deliver adjuvant chemotherapy? The role of postoperative adjuvant chemotherapy for soft tissue sarcomas is controversial, and may not be effective at all, as supported by recent survey and multicentric studies [69−71]. Nevertheless, preoperative chemotherapy identifies a selected group of responders who should be separately investigated, in terms of possible responders to adjuvant treatment, and for choice of effective therapy in the event of advanced disease.

The role of radiation therapy

It is still debatable whether radiotherapy should be employed before or after surgery. The enhancing effect of radiotherapy immediately after DX has already been clinically proved [18−20] and supports the rationale of the aforementioned protocol employed at UCLA [21, 29]: their results support the effect of this combined therapy, but the role of infusion itself was not verified. Our protocol, with surgery and pathologic evaluation immediately after infusion chemotherapy, documents that intra-arterial DX alone can achieve histologic necrosis, but not eradicate the tumor, and surgery or radiotherapy, or both, could provide proper local control. We consider it hazardous to rely only on intra-arterial chemotherapy plus radiotherapy. However, the possibility to achieve a long lasting local control even without surgery [14, 72] has been documented.

The role of HP

The survey on HP chemotherapy is even more confounding. The few reported studies have collected hundreds of cases, but data are not proportionally reliable. Limb-salvage philosophy is a basic intent of regional treatments, and evaluation of results can be subjective, however, not relying only on survival rate. Nevertheless, Krementz et al. [58], who studied 111 cases, reported an amazing five-year survival rate of 75−90%, but no other author has presented similar data, and it is difficult to compare series. Small recent reports [62, 63, 65] and ours agree with some common conclusions, which basically are: a) HP is effective on primary soft tissue sarcoma of the extremities, lowers the local recurrence rate but does not definitely eradicate the tumor, even if its level of tissue necrosis seems to be higher than after intra-arterial infusion, and should thus be included in a multimodality strategy; b) the survival rate of patients treated with HP chemotherapy is somehow related to the stage of disease; incidence of distant metastasis and mortality rate are not modified by HP; c) the choice of drugs to be used in HP is still to be defined.

Conclusions

In examining common points and differences between infusion and perfusion for soft tissue sarcomas, some general statements can be made. These preoperative regional treatments do not modify the disease-free interval, or overall survival [21, 35]. This is not surprising if we consider the non-significant results of postoperative adjuvant chemotherapy [69−71]. The effective role of regional treatments seems to be limited only to local control. Seventy percent of histologic necrosis >50% achieved by intra-arterial infusion and the possibility to improve these results with HP are unquestionably positive data, if only compared with the poor response rate of advanced sarcoma to chemotherapy [73]. Moreover, the pathologic necrosis provided by intra-arterial infusion is consistently found in the viable margins of the bulky tumor, and this observation is determinant in the judgement of adequacy after marginal operations, even in the presence of partial response. Improved staging systems, conservative surgical approaches, the better defined use of radiotherapy, and the documented effect of regional treatments that enhance results of surgery and radiotherapy have resulted in a drastic reduction of local recurrences, and it can now be stated that in most sarcomas of the extremi-

126

ties, amputation is not indicated from the clinical or ethical point of view. Almost all deaths from soft tissue sarcomas are a result of distant spread, and the cure rate can be improved by effective control of systemic disease, which is still being sought. The documented local control achieved by preoperative treatments and the possible related role of improved limb-sparing procedures are a reality. The still open questions should be investigated by experimental and clinical multicentric controlled studies.

References

1. Cantin, J., McNeer, G. P., Chu, F. C., Booher, R. J., 1968. The problem of recurrence after treatment of soft tissue sarcoma. Ann. Surg., 168: 47 – 53.
2. Lindberg, R. D., Marain, R. G., Romsdahl, M. M., Barkley, H. T., 1981. Conservative surgery and postoperative radiotherapy in 300 adults with soft-tissue sarcomas. Cancer, 47: 2391 – 2397.
3. Leibel, S. A., Tranbaugh, R. F., Wara, W. M., Becksted, J. H., Bovill, E. G. Jr., Phillips, T. L., 1982. Soft tissue sarcomas of the extremities. Survival and patterns of failure with conservative surgery and postoperative irradition compared to surgery alone. Cancer, 50: 1076 – 1083.
4. Chen, H. G., Gross, J. F., 1980. Intra-arterial infusion of anticancer drugs: theoretic aspects of drug delivery and review of responses. Cancer Treat. Rep., 64: 31 – 40.
5. Carlson, R. W., 1985. The rationale for continuous infusion scheduling of anticancer chemotherapy. EORTC Symposium on continuous infusion chemotherapy. Brussels, abstract no. 1.
6. Legha, S. S., Benjamin, R. S., Yap, H. Y., Freireich, E. J., 1979. Augmentation of adriamycin's therapeutic index by prolonged continuous i.v. infusion for advanced breast cancer. A. A. C. R., abstract no. 1059.
7. Legha, S. S., Benjamin, R. S., MacKay, B., Ewer, M., Wallace, S., Valdivieso, M., Rasmussen, S. L., Blumenschein, G. R., Freireich, E. J., 1982. Reduction of doxorubicin cardiotoxicity by prolonged continuous intravenous infusion. Ann. Intern. Med., 96: 133 – 139.
8. Swistel, A. J., Bading, J., Raaf, J. H., 1983. Comparison of intra-arterial versus intravenous adriamycin in the rabbit VX-2 tumor system. 36th Annual Symposium of the Society of Surgical Oncology, Denver, abstract, p. 54.
9. Tvete, S. T., Aaker Elsayed, E., Hope, A., Clausen, G., 1983. Uptake of adriamycin by sarcoma transplants in the rat kidney: Effects of renal arterial vs systemic constant rate infusion and of combination with ricin. Eur. J. Cancer Clin. Oncol., 19: 127 – 134.
10. Karakousis, C. P., Rao, U., Holtermann, O. A., Kanter, P. M., Holyoke, E. D., 1979. Tourniquet infusion chemotherapy in extremities with malignant lesions. Surg. Gynecol. Obstet., 149: 481 – 490.
11. Jönsson, P. E., Ingvar, C., Stridbeck, H., 1983. Tourniquet infusion with DTIC in therapy-resistant melanoma on the extremities: A pilot study. Recent Results Cancer Res., 86: 213 – 217.
12. Kantarjian, H. M., Bledin, A. G., Kim, E. E., Coçan, B. M., Chuang, V. P., Wallace, S., Haynie, T. P., 1983. Arterial perfusion with Tc-99m macroaggregated albumin (MAAAP) in monitoring intra-arterial chemotherapy of sarcomas. J. Nucl. Med., 24: 297 – 301.
13. Watkins, E. Jr., Sullivan, R .D., 1964. Cancer chemotherapy by prolonged arterial infusion. Surg. Gynecol. Obstet., 118: 3 – 19.
14. Marée, D., Bui, N. B., Chauvergne, J., Avril, A., Richaud, P., 1980. Traitment des sarcomes des tissus mous localement évolués. Intérêt de la chimiothérapie d'induction par voie intra-artérielle. Bull. Cancer (Paris), 67: 175 – 182.
15. Didolkar, M. S., Kanter, P. M., Baffi, R. R., Schwart, H. S., Lopez, R., Baez, N., 1978. Comparison of regional versus systemic chemotherapy with adriamycin. Ann. Surg., 187: 332 – 336.

16. Bern, M. M., McDermott, W., Cady, B., Oberfield, R. A., Trey, C., Clouse, M. E., Tullis, J. L., Parker, L. M., 1978. Intraarterial hepatic infusion and intravenous adriamycin for treatment of hepatocellular carcinoma. Cancer, 42: 399–405.

17. Lee, Y. N., Chan, K. K., Harris, P. A., Cohen, J. L., 1980. Distribution of adriamycin in cancer patients. Tissue uptakes, plasma concentration after iv and hepatic ia administration. Cancer, 45: 2231–2239.

18. Watring, W. G., Byfield, J. E., Lagasse, L. D., Lee, Y. D., Juillard, G., Jacobs, M., Smith, M. L., 1974. Combination adriamycin and radiation therapy in gynecologic cancer. Gynecol. Oncol., 2: 518–526.

19. Friedman, M., Afridi, M. A., Douglas, H. O. Jr., 1977. Simultaneous radiation and drug therapy: Tumor response and toxicity. J. Surg. Oncol., 9: 541–546.

20. Schaeffer, J., El-Mahdi, A. M., 1981. Combination adriamycin radiation treatment of pulmonary tumors in mice. Oncology, 38: 35–38.

21. Weisenburger, T. H., Eilber, F. R., Grant, T. T., Morton, D. L., Mirra, J. J., Steinberg, M., Rickles, D., 1981. Multidisciplinary 'limb salvage' treatment of soft tissue and skeletal sarcomas. Int. J. Radiat. Oncol. Biol. Phys., 7: 1495–1499.

22. Di Pietro, S., Gennari, L., 1964. Chemioterapia antiblastica regionale dei tumori del distretto cervico-facciale mediante infusione endoarteriosa continua. Tumori, 50: 267–308.

23. Di Pietro, S., De Palo, G. M., Gennari, L., Molinari, R., Damascelli, B., 1973. Cancer chemotherapy by intra-arterial infusion with adriamycin. J. Surg. Oncol. 5: 421–430.

24. Haskell, C. M., Eilber, F. R., Morton, D. L., 1975. Adriamycin (NSC-123127) by arterial infusion. Cancer Chemother. Rep., 6: 187–189.

25. Haskell, C. M., Silverstein, M. J., Rangel, D. M., Hunt, J. S., Sparks, F. C., Morton, D. L., 1974. Multimodality cancer therapy in man: A pilot study of adriamycin by arterial infusion. Cancer, 33: 1485–1490.

26. Morton, D. L., Eilber, F. R., Townsend, C. M. Jr., Grant, T. H., Mirra, J., Weisenburger, T. H., 1976. Limb salvage from a multidisciplinary treatment approach for skeletal and soft tissue sarcomas of the extremity. Ann. Surg. 184: 268–278.

27. Eilber, F. R., Mirra, J. J., Grant, T. T., Weisenburger, T. H., Morton, D. L., 1980. Is amputation necessary for sarcomas? A seven-year experience with limb salvage. Ann. Surg. 192: 431–438.

28. Eilber, F. R., Morton, D. L., Eckardt, J., Grant, T., Weisenburger, T. H., 1984. Limb salvage for skeletal and soft tissue sarcomas. Multidisciplinary preoperative therapy. Cancer 53: 2579–2584.

29. Eilber, F. R., Eckardt, J., Mirra, J., 1984. Preoperative intra-arterial adriamycin and radiation therapy for extremity, skeletal and soft tissue sarcomas. Symposium on intra-arterial and intracavitary chemotherapy, San Diego, abstract, pp. 101–104.

30. Kraybill, W. M., Harrison, M., Sasaki, T., Fletcher, W. S., 1977. Regional intraarterial infusion of adriamycin in the treatment of cancer. Surg. Gynecol. Obstet., 144: 335–338.

31. Karakousis, C. P., Lopez, R., Catane, R., Rao, U., Moore, T., Holyoke, E. D., 1980. Intraarterial adriamycin in the treatment of soft tissue sarcomas. J. Surg. Oncol., 13: 21–27.

32. Denton, J. W., Dunham, W. K., Salter, M., Urist, M. M., Balch, C. M., 1984. Preoperative regional chemotherapy and rapid-fraction irradiation for sarcomas of the soft tissue and bone. Surg. Gynecol. Obstet. 158: 545–551.

33. Mantravadi, R. V. P., Trippon, M. J., Patel, M. K., Walker, M. J., Das Gupta, T. K., 1984. Limb salvage in extremity soft-tissue sarcoma: combined modality therapy. Radiology, 152: 523–526.

34. Shuman, L. S., Chuang, V. P., Wallace, S., Benjamin, R. S., Murray, J., 1982. Intra-arterial chemotherapy of malignant fibrous histiocytoma of the pelvis. Radiology, 142: 343–346.

35. Azzarelli, A., Quagliuolo, V., Audisio, R. A., Bonfanti, G., Andreola, S., Gennari, L., 1983. Intra-arterial adriamycin followed by surgery for limb sarcomas. Preliminary report. Eur. J. Cancer Clin. Oncol., 19: 885–890.

36. Azzarelli, A., 1984. Preoperative intra-arterial chemotherapy (PIC) for soft tissue sarcomas of the extremities. Symposium on Management of Soft Tissue and Bone Sarcomas, Utrecht, abstract no. 10.

37. Russell, W. O., Cohen, J., Enzinger, F., Hajdu, S. I., Heise, H., Martin, R. G., Meissner, W., Miller, W. T., Schmitz, R. L., Suit, H. D., 1977. A clinical and pathological staging system for soft tissue sarcomas. Cancer, 40: 1562 – 1570.

38. Brenner, J., Magill, G. B., Sordillo, P. P., Cheng, E. W., Yagoda, A., 1982. Phase II trial of cisplatin (CPDD) in previously treated patients with advanced soft tissue sarcoma. Cancer, 50: 2031 – 2033.

39. Stephens, F. O., 1983. Pharmacokinetics of intra-arterial chemotherapy. Recent Results Cancer Res., 86: 1 – 12.

40. Busch, W., 1866. Über den einfluss, welche herptigene Erysipeln zuweilen auf organisierte neubildungen ausüben. Verh. Naturforsch. Preuss. Rhein Westphal., 23: 28 – 30.

41. Bruns, P., 1877. Die heilwirkung des Erysipels auf Geschwülste. Beitr. Klin. Chir., 3: 443 – 446.

42. Coley, W.B., 1893. The treatment of malignant tumors by repeated inoculation of erysipelas with a report of ten original cures. Am. J. Med. Sci., 105: 487 – 511.

43. Cavaliere, R., Ciocatto, S. C., Giovannella, B. C., Heidelberger, C., Johnson, R. O., Margottini, M., Mondovì, B., Moricca, G., Rossi-Fanelli, A., 1967. Selective heat sensitivity of cancer cells. Biochemical and clinical studies. Cancer, 20: 1351 – 1381.

44. Mondovì, B., Finazzi, Agrò, A., Rotilio, G., Strom, R., Moricca, G., Rossi Fanelli, A., 1969. The biochemical mechanism of selective heat sensitivity of cancer cells. II. Studies on nucleic acids and protein synthesis. Eur. J. Cancer, 5: 137 – 146.

45. Strom, R., Crifò, C., Rossi Fanelli, A., Mondovì, B., 1977. Selective heat sensitivity of cancer cells. Biochemical aspects of heat sensitivity of tumor cells. Recent Results Cancer Res., 59: 7 – 35.

46. Giovannella, B. C., Morgan, C. A., Stehlin, J. S., Williams, L., 1973. Selective lethal effect of supranormal temperatures on mouse sarcoma cells. Cancer Res., 33: 2568 – 2578.

47. Giovannella, B. C., Stehlin, J. S., Morgan, A. C., 1976. Selective lethal effect of supranormal temperatures on human neoplastic cells. Cancer Res., 36: 3944 – 3950.

48. Stehlin, J. S., Giovannella, B. C., de Ipolyi, L. R., Muenz, L., Anderson, R. F., 1975. Results of hyperthermic perfusion for melanoma of the extremities. Surg. Gynecol. Obstet., 140: 339 – 348.

49. Mikkelsen, R.B., Verma, S. P., Wallach, D. F. H., 1977. Hyperthemia and the membrane potential of erythrocyte membranes as studied by raman spectroscopy. In: Proceedings of the 2nd International Symposium, Essen, June 2 – 4. Urban and Schwarzenberg, Baltimore, pp. 160 – 162.

50. Hauzman, J., 1979. The pH of cytoplasm as an important factor in the survival of in vitro-cultured malignant cells after hyperthermia. Eur. J. Cancer 15: 1281 – 1288.

51. Dickson, J. A., Shah, S. A., 1972. The effect of hyperthermia (42 °C) on the biochemistry and growth of a malignant cell line. Eur. J. Cancer, 8: 561 – 571.

52. Dewey, W.C., Weitra, A., Miller, H. M., 1971. Heat-induced lethality and chromosomal damage in synchronized Chinese hamster cells treated with 5-bomo-deoxyuridine. Int. J. Radiol. Biol., 20: 505 – 515.

53. Weitra, A., Dewey, W. C., 1971. Variation in sensitivity to heat shock during the cell cycle of Chinese hamster cells 'in vitro'. Int. J. Radiat. Biol., 19: 467 – 477.

54. Goldenberg, D. M., Langnen, M., 1971. Direct and abscopal antitumor action of local hyperthermia. Z. Naturforsch., 266: 359 – 361.

55. Schecter, M., Stowe, S. M., Moroson, M., 1978. Effects of hyperthermia on primary and metastatic tumor growth and host immune response in rats. Cancer Res., 38: 498 – 502.

56. Hahn, G. M., 1978. Interactions of drugs and hyperthermia in vitro and in vivo. In: Cancer Therapy by Hyperthermia and Radiation, Urban and Schwarzenberg, Baltimore, p. 72.

57. Natali, P. G., Zupi, G., Greco, C., Cavaliere, R., Giacomini, P., Ferrone, S., 1983. Effect of

hyperthermia and antineoplastic drugs on cell survival and antigenic profile of two human melanoma cell lines (abstract no. 246). Proceedings 13th Int. Congress of Chemotherapy, Vienna.

58. Krementz, E. T., Muchmore, J. H., 1983. Soft Tissue Sarcomas: Behavior and Management. Year Book Medical, Chicago, pp. 147 – 196.

59. Karakousis, C. P., Kanter, P. M., Park, H. C., Sharma, S. D., Moore, R., Ewing, J. H., 1982. Tourniquet infusion versus hyperthermic perfusion. Cancer, 49: 850 – 858.

60. Stehlin, J. S. Jr., 1969. Hyperthermic perfusion with chemotherapy for cancers of the extremities. Surg. Gynecol. Obstet., 129: 305 – 308.

61. McBride, C. M., McMurtrey, M. J., Copeland, E. M., Hickey, R. C., 1978. Regional chemotherapy by isolation-perfusion. Int. Adv. Surg. Oncol., 1: 1 – 9.

62. Schraffordt Koops, H. S., Eibergen, R., Oldhoff, J., Van der Ploeg, E., Vermey, A., 1976. Isolated regional perfusion in the treatment of soft tissue sarcomas of the extremities. Clin. Oncol., 2: 245 – 252.

63. Lehti, P. M., Moseley, H. S., Peetz, M. E., Fletcher, W. S., 1982. Liposarcoma of the leg. Am. J. Surg., 144: 44 – 47.

64. Stehlin, J. S. Jr., de Ipolyi, P. D., Giovanella, B. C., Gutierrez, A. E., Anderson, R. F., 1975. Soft tissue sarcomas of the extremity. Multidisciplinary therapy employing hyperthermic perfusion. Am. J. Surg., 130: 643 – 649.

65. Braat, R. P., Wieberdink, J., van Slooten, E., Olthuis, G., 1983. Regional perfusion with adriamycin in soft tissue sarcomas. Recent Results Cancer Res., 86: 260 – 263.

66. Enneking, W.F., Spanier, S. S., Goodman, M. A., 1980. A system for the surgical staging of musculoskeletal sarcoma. Clin. Orthop., 153: 106 – 120.

67. Enneking, W. F., Spanier, S. S., Malawer, M. M., 1981. The effect of the anatomic setting on the results of surgical procedures for soft parts sarcoma of the thigh. Cancer, 47: 1005 – 1022.

68. Greene, R. F., Collins, J. M., Jenkins, J. F., Speyer, J. L., Myers, C. E., 1983. Plasma pharmacokinetics of adriamycin and adriamycinol: implications for the design of in vitro experiments and treatment protocols. Cancer Res., 43: 3417 – 3421.

69. Edmonson, J. H., Fleming, T. R., Ivins, J. C., Burgert, E. O., Soule, E. H., O'Connell, M. J., Sim, F. H., Ahmann, D. L., 1982. Randomized study of systemic chemotherapy following complete excision of non-osseous sarcomas: interim report. Proc. Am. Soc. Clin. Onc., 1: 182.

70. Antman, K., Suit, H., Amato, D., Corson, J., Wood, W., Proppe, K., Harmon, D., Carey, R., Greenberger, J., Blum, R., Wilson, R., 1983. Preliminary results of a randomized trial of adjuvant (ADJ) adriamycin (ADR) for sarcomas (S): lack of apparent difference between treatment groups. Proc. Am. Soc. Clin. Oncol., 2: 236.

71. Bramwell, V. H. C., Rouesse, J., Santoro, A., Buesa, J., Somers, R., Thomas, D., Sylvester, R., Pinedo, H. M., 1985. European experience of adjuvant chemotherapy for soft tissue sarcoma – a randomised trial comparing cyvadic with control (preliminary report). Cancer Treat. Rep., In press.

72. Mira, J. G., Chu, F. C. H., Fortner, J. G., 1977. The role of radiotherapy in the management of malignant hemangiopericytoma. Report of eleven new cases and review of the literature. Cancer, 39: 1254 – 1259.

73. Pinedo, H. M., Kenis, Y., 1977. Chemotherapy of advanced soft-tissue sarcomas in adults. Cancer Treat. Rev., 4: 67 – 86.

9. Phase II new drug trials in soft tissue sarcomas

Allan T. Van Oosterom

As stated in chapter 6, doxorubicin remains the most active single chemotherapeutic agent in the treatment of metastatic soft tissue sarcomas. Approximately 25% of the patients treated with Doxorubicin will have a clinical response [1–5]. This was demonstrated with an interval of ten years in the USA [2] and Europe [4, 5]. A steep dose response curve documented in several series [2, 5] led to the recommendation to give the drug in a dose just tolerated by the bone marrow. Further studies with combinations in which DTIC, Vincristine, Cyclophosphamide and/or Actinomycin D were included, depicted, however not in randomized trials, a survival advantage for responders to the combinations. Median survivals of 15 months versus 8 months were reported [6–8]. Alterations in the basic CYVADIC regimen (Table 1) have been conducted in an effort to increase response and survival and to reduce toxicity [9–11] but offered no advantage over the conventional 5-day regimen. The last study [11] however revealed that the performance status of the patients was the major prognostic determinant for response. This could also explain the wide differences in response rates reported in several series. The only progress with the combinations was the observation that in a subgroup of patients the application of surgery could render these patients free of disease and a survival advantage was observed [12]. Considering this minimal advantage with the combination it is not surprising that several cooperative groups – ECOG and EORTC – have continued to use single-agent Adriamycin as their 'standard' of comparison, for first line treatment.

From the data hitherto presented it is obvious that the final outcome for most patients with advanced soft tissue sarcomas remains dismal with less than a five percent chance of cure. This observation stresses the need to perform phase II studies with the anticipated result to discover new active drugs for the treatment of soft tissue sarcoma.

Phase II testing in sarcomas has been very disappointing as Samson reported in the previous edition of this volume [13]. In the recent past again a considerable amount of drugs (Table 2 and 3) have been tested in many patients resistant to Adriamycin alone and Adriamycin containing combinations.

Pinedo, H. M., Verweij, J (eds) Clinical Management of Soft Tissue Sarcomas
© *1986 Martinus Nijhoff Publishers, Boston. ISBN 0-89838-808-2. Printed in The Netherlands.*

Table 1.

Cyvadic regimen:		
Cyclophosphamide	600 mg/m²	d 1
Vincristin	1.2 mg/m²	d 1
Adriamycin	50 mg/m²	d 1
DTIC	250 mg/m²	d 1 – 5
	q 3 wks	

The Southwest Oncology Group tested subsequently Gallium Nitrate 700 mg/m² q 2 wks, which proved negative in 31 patients [14], and the combination of vincristine 1.0 mg/m² + high-dose methotrexate 5.0 g/m² with leucovorin rescue q 2 wks, which showed some activity, 2 partial responses in 14 patients. The authors describe however that they plan no further studies of this combination in adult patients with sarcomas [15]. A further study of the SWOG concerns Mitoxantrone 12mg/m² q 3 wks [16]. This anthraquinone derivative is devoid of activity, notwithstanding it's structural relationship with Adriamycin, only 1 partial response in 61 patients.

Other negative data about this drug are reported in a review by Smith [17]. The

Table 2. Recently tested inactive drugs in soft tissue sarcoma in all groups but the EORTC.

Drug	Group	N	CR	PR	Reference
Gallium nitrate	SWOG	31	1	1	[14]
Mitoxantrone	SWOG	61	–	1	[16]
Aziridinylbenzoquinone	SWOG	39	–	1	[18]
Dibromodulcitol	ECOG	45	–	1	[19]
ICRF-159	ECOG	37	–	1	[19]
Maytansine	ECOG	47	–	–	[19]
Cisplatinum	GOG	28	2	3	[20]
Cisplatinum	MSK	34	–	2	[21]
VP16-213	MSK	26	–	–	[25]
Metoprine	MSK	46	2	2	[26]
4 demethoxydaunorubicin	MSK	35	1	1	[27, 28]
Lonidamine	MSK	21	–	1	[29]
Vindesine cont. infusion	MDA	15	1	–	[30]
Vinblastine cont. infusion	MDA	15	–	–	[30]
Bisantrene	MDA	10	–	1	[31]
PALA	MDA	20	1	–	[32]
Chlorozotocin	WOMG	29	–	4	[34]

N   = Number of evaluable patients.
CR = Complete response.
PR = Partial response.

most recent report of the SWOG is about aziridinylbenzoquinone (AZQ), 40 mg/m^2 q 3 wks. Only one partial response was noted among 39 treated patients [18].

A further negative report came from the ECOG, which evaluated Dibromodulcitol 180 mg/m^2 p.o. days 1–10 every 4 wks, ICRF-159 300 mg/m^2 3 times daily orally, days 1–3 every 4 wks and maytansine 1.5 mg/m^2 intravenously q 3 wks [19]. Adequate numbers of patients were entered in all three studies but failed to show activity.

The Gynecologic Oncology Group tested cisplatinum 50 mg/m^2 q 3 wks in 28 evaluable patients with advanced mixed mesodermal sarcomas. Two complete and three partial responses (overall response rate 18%) were observed [20]. Several studies in the past with this drug were negative [21–23]. All patients in the GOG study were heavily pretreated, so mixed mesodermal sarcomas might constitute a special type where CDDP must be considered for inclusion into combinations. However, in other sarcoma types CDDP was found not active even in previously untreated patients [24]. Other drugs tested in Memorial Sloan-Kettering were VP-16-213 120 mg/m^2 d 1, 3, 5 q 3 wks, applied intravenously which appeared not to have significant activity [25] and metoprine 40–60 mg/m^2 orally every 22–3 wks, tested both in previously treated, but also in untreated, patients. Although some [26] activity was found in the pretreated group this could not be confirmed in the untreated group [24]. This group also tested 4-demethoxydaunorubicin 12.5 mg/m^2 q 3 wks, but found only one partial response in the 22 evaluable patients [27]. Tested in non-pretreated patients the drug did not show more activity [28]. Finally a study with lonidamine 430 mg/m^2 p.o. daily continuously up to 22 wks also did not show significant activity of this drug [29].

Table 3. Second line phase II studies of the EORTC soft tissue and bone sarcoma group.

Drug	N	PR	No change	Prog. arrest.	Reference
Cisplatin	17	–	4	23%	[23]
Chlorozotocin	17	–	3	18%	[35]
Methotrexate	26	–	4	15%	[36]
PALA	27	1	4	18%	[33]
Elliptinium	19	–	8	42%	[38]
Mitomycin C	34	–	12	37%	[37]
Cyclophosphamide	23	1	8	39%	[42]
Ifosfamide	21	1	12	62%	[42]

All studies but the last randomized one are closed to entry.

N = Number of evaluable patients.

PR = Practical response.

Prog. Arrest is defined as the sum of the responders and the no changes in the 6 weeks after the initiation of the treatment in patients progressive in the 6 weeks prior to entry.

Other negative studies were reported from the M. D. Anderson Group about continuous 5-day infusion of vindesine 1.2 mg/m^2/day q 3 wks and continuous infusion of vinblastine 1.5 mg/m^2/day $\times$ 5 q 3 wks [30], bisantrene 100 mg/m^2/day $\times$ 5 q 3 wks [31] and PALA 6 g/m^2 q 2 wks [32]; the latter drug was previously tested by the EORTC Group which did also not find activity [33].

Further confirmation about the ineffectivity of chlorozotocin could be derived from both a study, in which 150 mg/m^2 q 6 wks was given, reported by Presant [34] and a study of Mouridsen, who applied 120 mg/m^2 q 4 wks [35]. The EORTC Group further reported negative studies of low-dose methotrexate 40 mg/m^2 weekly [36], mitomycine C 12 mg/m^2 q 3 wks [37] and 9-hydroxy methyl elliptinium 100 mg/m^2 weekly [38].

The activity of fibroblast Interferon (HuIFN-B) was investigated in 20 pretreated patients and only minimal clinical benefit was observed [39]. As previously mentioned most patients selected for these phase II studies were pretreated. However, some groups also included non-pretreated patients and the results did not improve [24]. Analysis of the performance status as the major prognostic determinant for response in sarcomas did not reveal a difference between first and second line patients within the EORTC studies [46].

Further analysis of the data, however, revealed that where the EORTC standard phase II protocols ask for disease progression in the 6 weeks prior to entry, a progression arrest of over 50% in the patients entered might indicate activity of the drug if tested in first line treatment. The EORTC Group performed this, as will be reported later in this chapter [42]. Further proof for this progression arrest observation will be derived from an ongoing study in which Adriamycin 75 mg/m^2 is tested in patients who failed on first line non-Adriamycin containing regimens.

A drug with real activity can also be discovered in this classical Phase II study setting as was shown for Ifosfamide. This drug is the only positive discovery of the recent past and its effectivity has been reported by many groups [40–44]. The report of Stuart Harris [40] of 42 non-pretreated patients with different treatment schedules, 5.0–8.0 g/m^2 every 3 wks, and mesna rescue showed a 38 percent response rate but the toxicity encountered proved considerable. Scheulen et al., applying 60 mg/kg/day i.v. on five consecutive days every 3–4 wks, [41] observed five responses (2 CR, 3 PR) in sixteen evaluable pretreated patients (31%). The most remarkable observation in this study is the two responses in cyclophosphamide-refractory patients. The EORTC study in 121 evaluable patients and reported by Bramwell [42], randomized in pretreated and non-pretreated patients between Cyclophosphamide 1.5 g/m^2 and Ifosfamide 5.0 g/m^2 both every 3 wks. It confirmed the activity of Ifosfamide with another less toxic method of administration, suggested a higher response rate and less myelotoxicity for Ifosfamide over Cyclophosphamide, which may have advantages for inclusion into combinations. The higher response rate observed for females on Cyclophosphamide and for patients on Ifosfamide in Britain versus the Continent will be reexamined in the final analysis. Another 5-day regimen was reported by Magrath 1800 mg/m²/day × 5 q 3 wks [43] who also observed responses in cyclophosphamide-resistant patients, as will shortly be reported by Antman 2−2.5 g/m²/day × 4 q 3 wks [44]. Studies to determine the response rate of the combination of Adriamycin and Ifosfamide are in progress [45] and promising results have been obtained. The combination will be tested in comparison with Adriamycin alone. This drug remains the cornerstone of the treatment of advanced soft tissue sarcomas since randomized studies with Adriamycin analogs as Carminomycin [4] and 4-Epi-Adriamycin [5] have failed to show superiority of the newer analogs over Adriamycin.

From the data presented it can be derived that the search for new active drugs in soft tissue sarcoma must continue and should preferably be performed in patients with a good performance status. A drug showing activity in pretreated patients needs to be tested up-front.

References

1. Blum, R. H.: An overview of studies with Adriamycin (NSC 123127) in the United States. Cancer Chemother. Rep., 6: 247−251, 1975.
2. O'Bryan, R. M., Baker, L. H., Gottlieb, J. E., Rivkin, S. E., Balcerzak, S. P., Grumet, G. N., Salmon, S. E., Moon, T. E. and Hoogstraten, B.: Dose response evaluation of Adriamycin in human neoplasia. Cancer, 39: 1940−1948, 1977.
3. Schoenfeld, D. A., Rosenbaum, C., Horton, J., Wolter, J. M., Falkson, G. and DeConti, R. C.: A comparison of Adriamycin versus vincristine and Adriamycin, and cyclophosphamide versus vincristine, actinomycin D, and cyclophosphamide for advanced sarcoma. Cancer, 50: 2757−2762, 1982.
4. Bramwell, V. H. C., Mouridsen, H. T., Mulder, J. H., Somers, R., Van Oosterom, A. T., Santoro, A., Thomas, D., Sylvester, R., Markham, D.: Carminomycin vs. adriamycin in advanced soft tissue sarcomas; an EORTC randomized phase II study. Eur. J. Cancer Clin. Oncol. 19: 1097−1104, 1983.
5. Mouridsen, H. T., Somers, R., Santoro, A., Mulder, J. H., Bramwell, V., Van Oosterom, A. T., Sylvester, R., Thomas, D., Pinedo, H. M.: Doxorubicin vs epirubicin in advanced soft tissue sarcomas. An EORTC randomized phase II study. In: Advances in anthracycline chemotherapy: Epirubicin, edited by Bonadonna, G., Masson Milano, 95−103, 1984.
6. Gottlieb, J. A., Benjamin, R. S., Baker, L. H., O'Bryan, R. M., Rivkin, S. E. and Bodey, G. P.: Role of DTIC (NSC 45388) in the chemotherapy of sarcomas. Cancer Treatm. Rep., 60: 199−203, 1976.
7. Benjamin, R. S., Gottlieb, J. A., Baker, L. H. and Sinkovics, J. G.: CYVADIC vs. CYVADACT − A randomized trial of cyclophosphamide, vincristine, Adriamycin, plus dacarbazine, or actinomycin-D in metastatic sarcomas. Proc. AACR and ASCO, 17: 256, 1976.
8. Yap, B. S., Baker, L. H., Sinkovics, J. G., Rivkin, S. E., Bottomley, R., Thigpen, T., Burgess, M. A., Benjamin, R. S. and Bodey, G. P.: Cyclophosphamide, vincristine, Adriamycin, and DTIC (CYVADIC) combination chemotherapy for the treatment of advanced sarcomas. Cancer Treatm. Rep., 64: 93−98, 1980.
9. Benjamin, R. S. and Yap, B. S.: Infusion chemotherapy for soft tissue sarcomas. In: Soft Tissue Sarcomas, edited by Baker, L. H., Martinus Nijhoff Publishers, The Hague, The Netherlands, 1983.

10. Bernard, S. A., Capizzi, R. L., Rudnick, S. A., Tremont, S. J. and Raymond, R. N.: A one-day combination chemotherapy (CYVADIC) regimen in soft tissue sarcomas. Proc. ASCO, 1: 170, 1982.

11. Pinedo, H. M., Bramwell, V. H. C., Mouridsen, H. T., Somers, R., Vendrik, C. P. J., Santoro, A., Buesa, J., Wagener, Th., van Oosterom, A. T., van Unnik, J. A. M., Sylvester, R., de Pauw, M., Thomas, D. and Bonadonna, G.: Cyvadic in Advanced Soft Tissue Sarcoma: A randomized study comparing two schedules. Cancer 53: 1825 – 1832, 1984.

12. Yap, B. S., Sinkovics, J. G., Burgess, M. A., Benjamin, R. S. and Bodey, G. P.: The curability of advanced soft tissue sarcomas in adults with chemotherapy. Proc. ASCO, 2: 239, 1983.

13. Samson, M. K.: Phase II New Drug Trials in soft tissue sarcomas. In: Soft Tissue Sarcomas, edited by Baker, L. H.; Martinus Nijhoff Publishers, The Hague, The Netherlands: 135 – 140, 1983.

14. Saiki, J. H., Baker, L. H., Stephens, R. L., Fabian, C. J., Kraut, E. H. and Fletcher, W. S.: Gallium Nitrate in Advanced Soft Tissue and Bone Sarcomas: A Southwest Oncology Group Study. Cancer Treatm. Rep., 66: 1673 – 1674, 1982.

15. Vaughn, C. B., McKelvey, E., Balcerzak, S. P., Loh, K., Stephens, R. and Baker, L. H.: High-Dose Methotrexate With Leucovorin Rescue Plus Vincristine in Advanced Sarcoma: A Southwest Oncology Group Study. Cancer Treatm. Rep. 68: 409 – 410, 1984.

16. Bull, F. E., Von Hoff, D. D., Balcerzak, S. P., Stephens, R. L. and Panettiere, F. J.: Phase II Trial of Mitoxantrone in Advanced Sarcomas: A Southwest Oncology Group Study. Cancer Treatm. Rep. 69: 231 – 233, 1985.

17. Smith, I. E.: Mitoxantrone (novantrone): A review of experimental and early clinical studies. Cancer Treatm. Rev. 10: 103 – 115, 1983.

18. Zidar, B., Baker, L., Rivkin, S., Balcerzak, S., Stephens, R.: A Phase II Study of Aziridinylbenzoquinone (AZQ) in advanced soft tissue and bony sarcoma. A Southwest Oncology Group (SWOG) Study. Proc. ASCO, 4: 130, 1985.

19. Borden, E. C., Ash, A., Enterline, H. T., Rosenbaum, Ch., Laucius, J. F., Paul, A. R., Falkson, G., Lerner, H.: Phase II evaluation of dibromodulcitol, ICRF-159, and maytansine for sarcomas. Am. J. Clin. Oncol. (CCT) 5: 417 – 420, 1982.

20. Thigpen, T., Shingleton, H., Homesley, H. and Blessing, J., for the Gynecologic Oncology Group: Phase II trial of Cis-Diamminedichloroplatinum (DDP) in treatment of advanced or recurrent mixed mesodermal sarcoma of the uterus. Proc. ASCO, 1: 110, 1982.

21. Brenner, J., Magill, G. B., Sordillo, P. P., Cheng, E. W., Yagoda, A.: Phase II Trial of Cisplatin (CPDD) in Previously Treated Patients with Advanced Soft Tissue Sarcoma. Cancer 50: 2031 – 2033, 1982.

22. Samson, M. K., Baker, L. H., Benjamin, R. S., Lane, M., Plager, C.: Cisdichlorodiammineplatinum (II) in advanced soft tissue sarcomas: A Southwest Oncology Group Study. Cancer Treatm. Rep. 63: 2027 – 2029, 1979.

23. Bramwell, V. H. C., Brugarolas, A., Mouridsen, H. T., Cheix, F., de Jager, R., van Oosterom, A. T., Vendrik, C. P., Pinedo, H. M., Sylvester, R. and de Pauw, M.: EORTC phase II study of cisplatin in Cyvadic-resistant soft tissue sarcoma. Eur. J. Cancer 15: 1511 – 1513, 1979.

24. Magill, G. B.: Personal Communication, 1985.

25. Welt, S., Magill, G. B., Sordillo, P. P., Cheng, E., Hakes, T., Wittes, R. E. and Yagoda, A.: Phase II Trial of VP-16-213 in adults with advanced soft tissue sarcomas. Proc. ASCO, 2: 234, 1983.

26. Magill, G. B., Brenner, J., Sordillo, P. P., Cheng, E., Welt, W. and Currie, V. E.: Phase II trials of Metoprine (DDMP) in pretreated adults with advanced soft tissue sarcomas. Proc. ASCO, 1: 22, 1982.

27. Raymond, V., Magill, G. B., Welt, S., Kruger, G., Sordillo, P. P., Cheng, E. and Young, C. W.: 4-Demethoxydaunorubicin (DMDR) in advanced soft tissue sarcomas (STS): A Phase II Study. Proc. ASCO, 2: 235, 1983.

28. Wissel, P., Magill, G., Raymond, V., Welt, S., Sordillo, P. P. and Cheng, E.: 4'Demethoxydaunorubicin (DMDR) in advanced soft tissue sarcomas: An update with emphasis on patients (PTS) without prior doxorubicin (DOX). Proc. ASCO 3: 259, 1984.

29. Wissel, P., Magill, G., Welt, S., O'Hehir, M., Sordillo, P. and Currie, V.: Phase II Trial of Lonidamine (1,-2,4-Dichlorophenyl)-1H-Indazol-3-Carbollytic Acid) (LON) in advanced soft tissue sarcomas. Proc. ASCO 3: 258, 1984.

30. Yap, B. S., Benjamin, R. S., Plager, C., Burgess, M. A., Papadopoulos, N. and Bodey, G. P.: A randomized study of continuous infusion vindesine versus vinblastine in adults with refractory metastatic sarcomas. Am. J. Clin. Oncol. (CCT) 6: 235–238, 1983.

31. Papadopoulos, N. E. J., Tenney, D. M., Benjamin, R. S., Plager, C., Chawla, S. P., Yap, B. S., Bodey, G. P.: Phase II study of bisantrene in advanced sarcoma. Proc. ASCO 3: 264, 1984.

32. Kurzrock, R., Yap, B. S., Plager, C., Papadopoulos, N., Benjamin, R. S., Valdivieso, M., Bodey, G. P.: Phase II Evaluation of PALA in patients with refractory metastatic sarcomas. Am. J. Clin. Oncol. 7 (4): 305–307, 1984.

33. Bramwell, V., Van Oosterom, A. T., Mouridsen, H. T., Cheix, F., Somers, R., Thomas, D. and Rozencweig, M.: N-(Phosphonacetyl)-L-Aspartate (PALA) in advanced soft tissue sarcoma: A Phase II trial of the EORTC Soft Tissue Sarcoma Group. Eur. J. Cancer Clin. Oncol. 18 (1): 81–84, 1982.

34. Presant, C. A., Bartolucci, A. A.: Phase II evaluation of Chlorozotocin in metastatic sarcomas. Med. Pediatr. Oncol. 12: 25–27, 1984.

35. Mouridsen, H. T., Bramwell, V. H. C., Lacave, J., Metz, R., Vendrik, C. P. J., Hild, J., McCreanney, J. and Sylvester, R.: Treatment of advanced soft tissue sarcomas with chlorozotocin. A Phase II trial of the EORTC Soft Tissue and Bone Sarcoma Group. Cancer Treatm. Rep.: 509–511, 1981.

36. Buesa, J. M., Mouridsen, H. T., Bonadonna, G., Somers, R., van Oosterom, A. T., Jasmin, G., Bramwell, V., Cortes Funes, H., Vendrik, C. P. J., Wagener, T. and Thomas, D.: Treatment of advanced soft tissue sarcomas with low dose Methotrexate. A Phase II trial of the EORTC Soft Tissue and Bone Sarcoma Group. Cancer Treatm. Rep. 68: 683–684, 1984.

37. Van Oosterom, A. T., Santoro, A., Bramwell, V., Davy, M., Mouridsen, H. T., Thomas, D. and Sylvester, R.: Mitomycin C (MMC) in advanced soft tissue sarcoma: A Phase II Study of the EORTC Soft Tissue and Bone Sarcoma Group. Eur. J. Cancer Clin. Oncol. 21: 459–461, 1985.

38. Somers, R., Rouëssé, J., Van Oosterom, A. T. and Thomas, D.: Phase II study of Elliptinium in metastatic soft tissue sarcoma. Eur. J. Cancer and Clin. Oncol. 21: 591–593, 1985.

39. Harris, J. E., Das Gupta, T. and Vogelzang, N.: Treatment of soft tissue sarcoma with fibroblast interferon (HuIFN-B)-American Cancer Society/Illinois Cancer Council Study – Final Report. Proc. ASCO 4: 222, 1985.

40. Stuart-Harris, R. C., Harper, P. G., Parsons, C. A., Kaye, S.B., Mooney, C. A., Gowing, N. F. and Wiltshaw, E.: High-dose alkylation therapy using ifosfamide infusion with mesna in the treatment of adult advanced soft-tissue sarcoma. Cancer Chemother. Pharmacol. 11: 65–72, 1983.

41. Scheulen, M. E., Niederle, N., Bremer, K., Schütte, J. and Seeber, S.: Efficacy of ifosfamide in refractory malignant diseases and uroprotection by mesna: Results of a clinical phase II-study with 151 patients. Cancer Treatm. Rev. 10, (Suppl. A): 93–101, 1983.

42. Bramwell, V., Mouridsen, H., Santoro, A., Blackledge, G., Somers, R., Thomas, D., Sylvester, R., Bush, H.: Cyclophosphamide (CP) vs Ifosfamide (IF): A randomized phase II trial in adult soft tissue sarcoma (STS). Preliminary report of EORTC Soft Tissue and Bone Sarcoma Group. Proc. ASCO 4: 143, 1985.

43. Magrath, I. T., Sandlund, J.T., Rayner, A., Rosenberg, S. A., Arasi, V. and Miser, J. S.: Treatment of recurrent sarcomas with Ifosfamide (IF). Proc. ASCO 4: 136, 1985.

44. Antman, K. H., Montella, D., Rosenbaum, Ch. and Schwen, M.: A Phase II Trial of Ifosfamide

with Mesna in Previously Treated Metastatic Sarcoma. Cancer Treatm. Rep., 69: 499–504, 1985.

45. Schütte, J., Dombernowsky, P., Santoro, A., Steward, W., Mouridsen, H. T., Somers, R., van Oosterom, A. T., Blackledge, G., Thomas, D. and Sylvester, R.: Adriamycine (A) and Ifosfamide (I), A New Effective Combination in Advanced Soft Tissue Sarcoma. Proc. ASCO 5: 145, 1986.

46. Van Oosterom, A. T., Bramwell, V. H. C., Mouridsen, H. T., Somers, R., Santoro, A., Buesa, J., Vendrik, C. P., Rouëssé, J., Dombernowsky, P., Pinedo, H. M., Thomas, D. and Sylvester, R.: Review of the EORTC Soft Tissue and Bone Sarcoma Groups' Phase II Studies in Advanced Soft tissue sarcomas, Ed. J. van Unnik and A. T. van Oosterom, EORTC Monograph, Raven Press New York, 161–167, 1986.

Subject index